NHS Jargon Explained

NHS Jargon Explained

TONY WHITE
PhD FRCS MB BS AKC
Consultant Otolaryngologist (retired)

Foreword by
SIR IAN CARRUTHERS
Chief Executive
South West Strategic Health Authority

Radcliffe Publishing
Oxford • New York

Radcliffe Publishing Ltd
18 Marcham Road
Abingdon
Oxon OX14 1AA
United Kingdom

www.radcliffepublishing.com
Electronic catalogue and worldwide online ordering facility.

British Library Cataloguing in Publication Data
A catalogue record for this book is available from the British Library.

ISBN-13: 978 184619 469 6

The paper used for the text pages of this
book is FSC certified. FSC (The Forest
Stewardship Council) is an international
network to promote responsible
management of the world's forests.

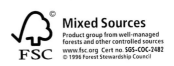

Mixed Sources
Product group from well-managed
forests and other controlled sources
www.fsc.org Cert no. SGS-COC-2482
© 1996 Forest Stewardship Council

FSC

Typeset by Pindar NZ, Auckland, New Zealand
Printed and bound by TJI Digital, Padstow, Cornwall, UK

Contents

Foreword

When it comes to navigating our way around the health service, those of us working in the NHS are only too well aware of how we can suddenly become aware of gaps in our knowledge in such a fast moving environment.

This is a reflection of the constant rigours of change and improvement. The persistent pace of change has been a challenging feature of the NHS throughout its 62-year history.

I personally see such resilient flexibility and determined self-improvement as one of the greatest strengths of our modern health service.

As the NHS continues to become more open and transparent there is no more important time than now to have a quick reference guide that enables the greatest number of people to quickly come to terms with the language of the health service.

Our time-poor culture demands ever faster yet better information so I welcome this book for being both comprehensive and concise, making it the quick guide so many of us need to fully appreciate the workings of our greatly admired National Health Service.

Sir Ian Carruthers
Chief Executive
South West Strategic Health Authority
August 2010

Preface

I often meet doctors, nurses and others working in the health services who express a wish that they had received a broader range of non-clinical information earlier in their careers. Others who are committed to continuing professional development seek learning material that will enable them to handle the wider issues they confront on a day-to-day basis, and for which initial education failed to prepare them. Many trainers can also find it difficult to access a single source that provides material for non-clinical training. *The Doctor's Handbook* was written to address these and other needs revealed by research. Since publication there has been positive feedback received from specialist trainees and other grades of doctors, including many consultants and, surprisingly, NHS managers.

At the same time there remained other groups where certain sections of the original *Doctor's Handbook* were not required. The sections likely to appeal to these groups have therefore been published separately as *A Guide to the NHS* (to include the structure and organisation of the NHS, and health-related Acts, Reports, Guidance Notes and Codes of Conduct) and *NHS Jargon Explained* (to include the glossary of NHS terms and acronyms). Both books provide information not only to workers in the NHS at all levels, but also to managers and staff of commercial companies working with the NHS, and campaigners, patient interest groups, researchers and journalists who wish to understand it better.

As time passes further changes in the structure, funding and governance of the NHS continue and Acts, Reports and acronyms are added constantly, so with these more compact books the task of keeping things up to date will be made easier. Where possible, readers are guided to original sources for the latest information that is often readily available on various websites.

You will find this small book valuable in your current role and a quick source of useful information and support.

Tony White
August 2010

About the author

Tony White is a retired consultant otolaryngologist appointed in Bath, where he was clinical director for seven years. He has a PhD from Bath University with a thesis on 'The Role of Doctors in Management'.

Together with John Gatrell he undertook a three-year research project into the non-clinical development needs of doctors that resulted in publication of the NHS Training Directorate report, *Medical Student to Medical Director*.

He has written several books on medical management and contributed to and edited several other textbooks as well as writing numerous papers. He has lectured widely and organised many workshops on doctors' management development issues. He was a member of a number of national advisory committees to develop doctors' non-clinical skills and acted as regular tutor on training courses in various regions.

NHS Jargon Explained

Glossary of NHS terminology

The aim of this chapter is to provide you with information on useful terms and a glossary of health service, management, non-clinical and medico-legal terms along with some definitions. For clinicians some of the terminology might already be familiar.

I'm afraid that further new terms continue to be introduced, many related to new information technology. Some are fairly obvious and have been included not just for the sake of completeness but just in case they need clarification. Beware – quite often they are terms that have only a loose connection with their real meaning. You may need to check this out when you hear the expressions, but do not be surprised if the speaker is not aware of the correct meaning. The meaning may also relate to a specific connection. A few terms are attempts that have been made to transfer manufacturing terminology to medical work.

Abduction In clinical terms a form of logical inference, commonly applied in the process of medical diagnosis. Given an observation, abduction generates all known causes. (*See also* deduction, induction and inference.)

Absenteeism   Absence from work not authorised through appropriate channels.

Access rate   An estimate of the availability of facilities to people living in an identified locality, irrespective of where they are treated. The measure is stated as discharges and deaths per 1000 population.

Accident   Any unexpected or unforeseen occurrence, especially one that results in injury or damage.

Accident and Emergency (A&E)   The title given to the hospital department previously termed 'Casualty' and now frequently called 'Emergency'. The Accident and Emergency patient may be brought by ambulance or car, or may arrive on foot.

Accident report   A written report of an accident. The format of the report is laid down in health and safety legislation.

Accommodation (children)   Being provided with accommodation replaces the old voluntary care concept. It refers to a service that the local authority provides for the parents of children in need, and for their children. A child is not in care when they are being provided with accommodation. Nevertheless, the local authority has a number of duties towards children for whom it is providing accommodation, including the duty to discover the child's wishes regarding the provision of accommodation, and to give them proper consideration.

Accountability   Being answerable for one's decisions and actions. Accountability cannot be delegated.

Added value   A measure of productivity expressed in terms of the financial value of an item as a result of workforce. Often used loosely in the NHS.

Adolescents   Young people in the process of moving from childhood to adulthood. Because of their age, adolescents may have special needs as patients.

Adoption   Total transfer of parental responsibility from the child's natural parents to the adopters.

Advance care planning   The process of discussing the treatment and care a patient would or would not wish to receive in the event that they lose capacity to decide or are unable to express a preference. This might include their preferred place of care and who they would like to be involved in making decisions on their behalf.

Advance decision (England and Wales) or advance directive (Scotland)   A statement of a patient's wish to refuse a particular treatment or care if they become unable to make or communicate decisions for themselves. A valid advance refusal if applicable to the patient's current situation must be respected and is legally binding on those providing care in England and Wales (provided it relates to life-prolonging treatment and it satisfies the additional legal criteria). This is likely to become legally binding in Scotland and Northern Ireland.

Advance statement A statement of a patient's views about how they would or would not wish to be treated if they become unable to make or communicate decisions for themselves. This can be general and would involve considerations regarding their place of residence, religious and cultural beliefs along with other personal values and preferences, as well as their medical treatment and care.

Adversarial One of two kinds of court process: adversarial and inquisitorial. The adversarial system refers to a court process in which the parties bring competing claims so that the court decides the outcome on the merits of each case.

Advocate An individual acting on behalf of, and in the interests of, patients who may feel unable to represent themselves in their contacts with a healthcare or other facility.

Advisory boards Bodies established to ensure the National Programme for IT engages with stakeholders, such as patients, the public, and health and care professionals.

Affidavit Statement in writing and an oath sworn before a person who has the authority to administer it, e.g. a solicitor.

Amenity bed A bed in a single room or small NHS hospital ward for which a patient may be charged a small fixed amount for the hotel part of the cost, but not the cost of treatment, under section 12 of the 1977 NHS Act.

Analysis of expenditure by client group Analysis of expenditure over broad groups of service related to patient care groups, e.g. services for mentally ill people, services mainly for children, and general and acute hospital and maternity services.

- **Functional (objective):** The object for which the payment has been made – medical staff services, nursing staff services, transport services and so on.
- **Subjective:** According to the nature of the payment, e.g. salaries and wages, travel, drugs, etc.

Annual report A report, written annually, which details progress over the last year and plans for the following year. Includes financial and activity statements.

Apology A sincere expression of regret.

Appeal (Care of Child) Appeals in care proceedings are now to be heard by the High Court or, where applicable, the Court of Appeal. All parties to the proceedings will have equal rights of appeal. On hearing an appeal, the High Court can make such orders as may be necessary to give effect to its decision.

Application In computer technology this is a synonym for a program that carries out a specific type of task. Word processors or spreadsheets are common applications available on personal computers.

Arbitration The process of settling a disagreement between two or more parties by the introduction of an external body or person with authority to make and implement an agreement.

Arden syntax A language created to encode actions within a clinical protocol into a set of situation-action rules for computer interpretation, and also to facilitate exchange between different institutions.

Area Child Protection Committee (ACPC) Based on the boundaries of the local authority, it provides a forum for developing, monitoring and reviewing the local child protection policies, and promoting effective and harmonious co-operation between the various agencies involved. Although there is some variation from area to area, each committee is made up of representatives of the key agencies, who have authority to speak and act on their agency's behalf. ACPCs issue guidelines about procedures, tackle significant issues that arise, offer advice about the conduct of cases in general, make policy and review progress on prevention, and oversee interagency training.

Artificial intelligence (AI) Any artefact, whether embodied solely in computer software or a physical structure like a robot, that exhibits behaviours associated with human intelligence. (*See also* Turing test.)

Artificial intelligence in medicine The application of artificial intelligence methods to solve problems in medicine, e.g. developing expert systems to assist with diagnosis or therapy planning. (*See also* artificial intelligence and expert systems.)

Assessment Process by which the capacities and incapacities of people who may require community care are established by social services departments, with appropriate services thereby identified.

Assessment (children) Process of gathering together and evaluating information about a child, its family and circumstances. Its purpose is to determine children's needs, in order to plan for their immediate and long-term care and decide what services and resources must be provided. Childcare assessments are usually co-ordinated by social services, but depend on teamwork with other agencies (such as education and health).

Associates   Salaried doctors who support principals in hard-pressed areas, such as the London Implementation Zone Education Initiative area or remote parts of Scotland.

Asynchronous communication   Communication between two parties when the exchange does not require both to be an active participant in the conversation at the same time, e.g. sending a letter. (*See also* synchronous communication and email.)

Audit   Originally the process by which the probity of operations and activities of an organisation was examined (internal audit) and a report on the annual accounts produced (external audit). Now used more widely, e.g. clinical audit evaluates the effectiveness of clinical activities; and management audit evaluates the effectiveness and efficiency of organisational and management arrangements. It involves the process of setting or adopting standards and measuring performance against those standards, with the aim of identifying both good and bad practice and implementing changes to achieve unmet standards.

Audit Committee   A committee of an NHS trust or authority board, comprising non-executive members, which ensures probity in the corporate governance of the organisation. Following the Cadbury Report, NHS bodies should have such a body.

Audit trails   Anyone accessing a patient's record using the NHS Care Records Service is automatically recorded in an audit trail. This is like an electronic footprint that shows who they are, when they accessed the record and what they did.

Authorised person (children)   In relation to care and supervision proceedings, this is a person not from the local authority who is authorised by the Secretary of State to bring proceedings under section 31 of the Act. This covers the National Society for the Prevention of Cruelty to Children (NSPCC) and its officers. Elsewhere in the Act there is a reference to persons who are authorised to carry out specified functions, e.g. to enter and inspect independent schools.

Average daily available beds   The average number of staffed beds in each department in which patients are being treated, or could be treated, each day without any changes being made in facilities or staff. Beds borrowed from other departments are included.

Average length of stay The average number of days a bed is occupied by each patient.

Bayes' theorem Theorem used to calculate the relative probability of an event given the probabilities of associated events. Used to calculate the probability of a disease given the frequencies of symptoms and signs within the disease and within the normal population.

Bed bureau An administrative unit that ensures that patients needing urgent admission are directed to a hospital which will admit them.

Bed days

> ‣ **Available bed days:** the sum of beds available for use each day during a specified period of time.

> ‣ **Occupied bed days:** the sum of the number of beds occupied by patients each day during a specified period of time. This total, divided by the number of discharges and deaths during the same period, gives the average length of stay.

> ‣ **Vacant bed days:** the number obtained when the total of occupied bed days is subtracted from the available bed days.

Bed norm A measure of the bed requirements for a given population, expressed as number of beds per 1000 people. Bed norms may be used in several different ways: age specific, as in the case of hospital accommodation for the elderly – 10 beds per 1000 aged 65 years and over; or by specialty, as in the case of orthopaedic beds – 0.35 per 1000.

Bed occupancy The number of beds occupied by patients at a particular time, usually midnight. It may be expressed as a percentage of available beds.

Bed state The number of beds, both occupied and vacant, at a particular time.

Bed turnover The average number of patients using each bed in a given period, such as a year.

Behavioural science The study of individuals and groups in a working environment. Issues may include communication, motivation, organisational structure and organisational change. The science is still being developed and relies on contributions from psychology and sociology.

Benchmarking Defined by the UK Benchmarking Centre (1993) as the continuous, systematic search for best practices, and the implementation that will lead to superior performance.

Benchmarks Benchmarks are sources of information (e.g. cost, quality outcomes, etc.) used as comparators to compare perform-ance between similar organisations or systems.

Booked case   An elective admission where the date has been arranged in advance with the patient. Waiting lists should include booked cases.

British Association of Medical Managers (BAMM)   Aims to 'support the provision of quality healthcare by improving and supporting the contribution of doctors in management, together with all other activities which contribute to, further, or are ancillary to this principal aim'.

Broadband   A type of data transmission in which a single (telephone) wire can carry several channels at once. Cable TV, for example, uses broadband transmission.

Budget   A statement of the financial resources made available to a budget holder to provide an agreed level of service over a set period of time.

Business plan   A plan setting out the goals of an organisation and identifying the resources and actions needed to achieve them. Usually prepared on an annual basis, the business plan seeks to balance planned activity with income so as to minimise financial risk.

Caldicott Guardian   The member of staff in an NHS organisation who is responsible for ensuring that patient rights to confidentiality are protected.

Capacity   The ability to make a decision. An adult is deemed to have capacity unless, having been given all appropriate help and sup-port, it is clear that they cannot understand, retain, use or weigh up the information needed to make a particular decision or to communicate their wishes.

Capital asset   Land, property, plant or equipment valued at more than £5000.

Capital Asset Register   A list of all the capital assets of an organisation. This contains information required to administer a capital asset replacement programme such as the purchase price, acquisition and replacement date of assets.

Capital Asset Replacement Programme   A programme which uses depreciation accounting techniques to spread the cost of the replacement of capital assets.

Capital charges   Since 1991, the use/ownership of capital in the NHS has incurred a cost, the capital charge. This was introduced so that NHS capital was no longer regarded as a free good or gift from the state. Capital charges consist of two elements: depreciation and interest on fixed assets. The interest rate currently applied is 6%. NHS trusts retain depreciation charges within the trust and are required to make a target rate of return equivalent to the interest rate.

Capital programme   A plan over a period of time (normally five years) showing costs and starting and final dates of schemes of work to be charged to the capital allocation.

Career advice   Providing information on career opportunities and training requirements.

Career counselling   Discussing career options for which the individual may be most suited.

Care order (children)   Order made by the court under s31 (1)(a) of the Children Act placing the child in the care of the designated local authority. A care order includes an interim care order except where express provision to the contrary is made.

Care pathway   An approach to managing a specific disease or clinical condition that identifies what interventions are required, and sets out the various stages of care through which a patient passes and the expected outcome of treatment.

Care plan   A written statement of community care services to be provided following assessment (q.v.). The document details the care and treatment that a patient receives and identifies who delivers the care and treatment. This term covers the term 'individual plan' (*See also* health record).

Care Programme Approach (CPA)   The individual packages of care (care programmes), developed in conjunction with social services, for all patients accepted by the specialist psychiatric services. Care programmes may range from 'minimal' single-worker assessment and monitoring for individuals with less severe mental health and social needs, to complex and multi-professional assessments and treatment.

Care Record Development Board (CRDB)   Established as an independent body to provide advice to NHS Connecting for Health on a variety of issues arising from the development of the NHS Care Records Service. The CRDB was replaced on 1 October 2007 by the National Information Governance Board for Health and Social Care, which will continue to publish and review the NHS Care Record Guarantee, formerly produced by the CRDB (*See also* National Information Governance Board for Health and Social Care).

Care Record Guarantee   The commitment of the NHS in England to patients that it will use records about them in ways that respect their rights and promote their health and well-being. The Guarantee covers people's access to their own records, controls on others' access, how access will be monitored and policed, options to further limit access, access in an emergency and what happens when someone cannot make decisions for him or herself.

Carer   A person who regularly provides help (without pay) to someone who requires domestic, physical, emotional or personal care as a result of illness or disability. This term also incorporates friends, relatives and partners. There are thought to be six million 'informal carers'.

Case-based reasoning   An approach to computer reasoning that uses knowledge from a library of similar cases, rather than by accessing a knowledge base containing more generalised knowledge, such as a set of rules. (*See also* artificial intelligence and expert system.)

Case conference (children)   Formal meeting attended by representatives from all the agencies concerned with the child's welfare. This increasingly includes the child's parents (and the Act promotes this practice).

Casemix   The mixture of clinical conditions and severity of condition encountered in a particular healthcare setting.

Cash limit   A limit imposed by the government on the amount of cash a public body may spend during a given financial year. Separate cash limits may be set for revenue and capital.

Causal reasoning   A form of reasoning based on following from cause to effect, in contrast to other methods in which the connection is weaker, such as probabilistic association.

Chairman (chairperson or chair is more politically correct)   A person who leads or conducts discussions. A chair's skill and technique may be used in a one-to-one meeting or by indirect communication methods, such as the telephone.

Change agent   A third party, who may be a trained behavioural scientist, and who acts as a catalyst in bringing about change by means of an organisation development programme.

Checklist   A means of recording observations relating to fixed criteria; used to check compliance with agreed procedures or standards.

Child   A person under the age of 18 years. There is an important exception to this in the case of an application for financial relief by a 'child' who has reached 18 years and is, or will be, receiving education or training.

Child assessment order   The order requires any person who can do so to produce the child for an assessment and to comply with the terms of the order.

Child Protection Register   Central record of all children in a given area for whom support is being provided via inter-agency planning. Generally, these are children considered to be at risk of abuse or neglect. The register is usually maintained and run by social service departments under the responsibility of a custodian (an experienced social worker able to provide advice to any professional making inquiries about the child). Registration for each child is reviewed every six months.

Child minder   Person who looks after one or more children under the age of eight for reward, for more than two hours in any one day.

Children in need   A child is in need if: (a) he or she is unlikely to achieve or maintain (or have the opportunity of achieving or maintaining) a reasonable standard of health or development without the provision for him or her of services by a local authority; or (b) his or her health or development is likely to be significantly impaired (or further impaired) without the provision for him or her of such services; or (c) he or she is disabled.

Children living away from home   Children who are not being looked after by the local authority but are nevertheless living away from home, e.g. children in independent schools. The local authority has a number of duties towards such children, e.g. to take reasonably practicable steps to ensure that their welfare is being adequately safeguarded and promoted.

Choice   Giving patients more choice about how, when and where they receive treatment is one cornerstone of the government's health policy. In the context of NHS reforms, this is the overarching policy term given to range of initiatives within the reform of the NHS designed to act as a driver for efficiency, quality and effectiveness.

Choose and Book   Allows a patient, in partnership with health and care professionals, to book first outpatient appointments at the most appropriate date, time and place for the patient.

Clinic session   A session held, and not merely scheduled, for, by or on behalf of one consultant, senior hospital medical officer or dental officer. Now extended to include sessions run by nurses and other clinical staff.

Clinical budgeting   The allocation of specific budgets to consultant clinical staff who are responsible for the budget management. A part of management budgeting.

Clinical directorate   A unit of management for specific clinical services. A clinical directorate is usually led by a clinical director, who is often a consultant working in that role for a number of sessions per week. They are supported by a nurse and/or business manager. The extent to which management responsibilities for budgets and staff are devolved to directorates varies.

Clinical guideline   An agreed set of steps to be taken in the management of a clinical condition.

Clinical pathway   *See* clinical guideline.

Clinical protocol   *See* clinical guideline.

Clinical responsibilities   Range of activities for which a clinician is accountable.

Clinical Risk and Safety Board   Local NHS boards responsible for establishing a framework for the safe implementation and continuing use of new IT systems in local NHS organisations. The board is made up of clinical representatives including doctors, nurses and other healthcare professionals.

Clinical Spine Application (CSA)   The web-based application that enables healthcare professionals who do not have access to local NHS Care Records Service systems and services to have controlled access to the Personal Demographics Service (PDS) and the Personal Spine Information Service (PSIS). It enables clinicians and other staff to access information held on the Spine.

Clinician   Health professional such as a doctor or nurse, involved in clinical practice.

Clinician's sealed envelope   *See* sealing.

Closed beds   Beds which have not been used (i.e. closed) for longer than one month for the purpose of redecoration or structural alterations, or because of a shortage of staff, but are scheduled to be reopened at a future date.

Code   In medical terminological systems, the unique numerical identifier associated with a medical concept, which may be associated with a variety of terms, all with the same meaning. (*See also* term.)

Cognitive map   A process of recording information in related groupings and intended to assist lateral thinking. (*See also* mind map.)

Cognitive science   A multidisciplinary field studying human cognitive processes, including their relationship to technologically embodied models of cognition. (*See also* artificial intelligence.)

Commissioner   An organisation or individual involved in purchasing healthcare. (*See also* purchaser.)

Commissioning   Relates to the purchasing and contracting of healthcare services. It is a broad term that can cover a range of activities but in principle a distinction can be drawn between two levels of commissioning. At one level, commissioning can involve service planning and design, through identifying population need; assessing the local priorities; understanding the market; and determining where and how services should be provided and by whom. On another level, commissioning can involve the daily purchasing of services, through managing contracts and spending budgets.

Commissioning a patient-led NHS   The letter and attachments (entitled *Commissioning a Patient-led NHS*) was sent to NHS Chief Executives and others at the end of July 2005. It builds on the *NHS Improvement Plan* and *Creating a Patient-Led NHS*. The details contained in the papers relate to the form and function of primary care trusts and strategic health authorities and was designed to begin to address the tension between providing services and commissioning services in PCTs. It was also intended to prompt cost savings of £250 million; deliver practice-based commissioning (PBC) by December 2006 at the latest; and SHAs will be reconfigured to move towards alignment with Government Office boundaries.

Communication   The two-way process of exchanging ideas, thoughts, feelings and facts.

Communication strategy   A written statement of objectives for effective communication and a plan for meeting those objectives. The strategy should be consistent with the business plan.

Community care   The assessment and commissioning of health and social care and treatment to patients/clients outside hospital, who have an identified physical or mental illness or disability. It is often more narrowly associated with patients being resettled from institutional care, e.g. from large psychiatric hospitals, or frail, elderly people who previously would have remained in hospital care.

Community Health Councils (CHCs)   'Patient watchdog' bodies established as part of the NHS reorganisation in 1974. Their role included assisting with complaints and visiting NHS premises. The government published the *NHS Plan for England* in 2000, which proposed the abolition of CHCs in England and their replacement by Patient and Public Involvement Forums and Patient Advocate and Liaison Services and established by each NHS trust, including primary care trusts in England. CHCs have been retained in Wales and Scotland.

Community health services   These divide into two main groups:

patient care in the community – the treatment or care (outside hospital) of patients with identified physical or mental illness or disability; and services to the community – services of prevention or intervention that are provided to a population, such as immunisation, screening and health promotion.

Complainant   A person who expresses dissatisfaction. They may or may not be the patient concerned.

Complaint   An expression of dissatisfaction.

Complaints procedure (children)   The procedure that a local authority must set up in order to hear representations regarding the provision of services under Part III of the Children Act from a number of persons, including the child, the parents and 'such other person' as the authority considers has sufficient interest in the child's welfare to warrant his or her representations being considered by them.

Compliment   An expression of approval or satisfaction.

Computer-based patient record   *See* electronic medical record.

Computerised protocol   Clinical guideline or protocol stored on a computer system so that it may be easily accessed or manipulated to support the delivery of care. (*See also* clinical guideline.)

Computer Sciences Corporation (CSC)   The Local Service Provider (LSP) for the North West and West Midlands Cluster and North East and Eastern Clusters, delivering software developed by its main subcontractor iSoft.

Conciliation   The process of a layperson assisting two parties in dispute to reach informal agreement through discussion and persuasion without any legally binding status.

Conciliatory   The application of conciliation techniques particularly outside a formal conciliation process.

Concurrent jurisdiction (children)   The High Court, a County Court and a Magistrates' Court (Family Proceedings Court) all have jurisdiction to hear proceedings under the Children's Act.

Connectionism   The study of the theory and application of neural networks. (*See also* neural network.)

Consent to share   Where a patient has explicitly consented to share information across organisations for the purpose of their healthcare, or has expressed no preference so consent is inferred. The sharing of information will be on a need-to-know basis. A Summary Care Record exists and is visible to an authorised user with a legitimate relationship to the patient. Consent may be given in two ways.

- **Implied consent:** When a patient has not expressed a preference so consent to share is inferred. For example, when a GP sends clinical information to a consultant following a patient referral to specialist care, the GP is assuming the patient's consent to send that information as part of the referral.
- **Express consent:** When a patient expresses permission for the sharing of their clinical information across NHS organisations.

Patients may also express dissent to the sharing of information.

- **Dissent to share:** Prevents confidential information maintained by one legal organisation being accessible by another legal organisation, unless the information is sent as part of a direct clinical communication like a referral or discharge note. A Summary Care Record will exist but will not be automatically visible to any authorised user, when combined with Consent to Store.

Constant prices   A mechanism for comparing prices for goods and services over a number of years, which compensates for the distortion introduced by inflation.

Contact order (children)   Order requiring the person with whom a child lives, or is to live, to allow the child to visit or stay with the person named in the order.

Continuing education   Activities which provide education and training for staff. These may be used to prepare for specialisation or career development as well as facilitating personal development.

Continuing professional development (CPD)   Defined as: 'A process of lifelong learning for all individuals and teams which enables professionals to expand and fulfil their potential and which also meets the needs of patients and delivers the health and healthcare priorities of the NHS'.

Contract/Agreement   A document agreed between providers and purchasers of healthcare. Details activity, financial and quality levels to be achieved.

Contract currencies   Agreed units of measurement for contracting, e.g. finished consultant episodes.

Contracts   The basis for agreement on the services that should be provided to patients, including specification of quality. Block contracts specify facilities to be provided, and may include workload agreements including patient activity targets within an agreed range. Cost and volume contracts specify the level of services required by the purchaser. Purchasers can link payment with agreed activity. Provider units will be able to match funding with workload and deploy resources more flexibly. Cost per case contracts cover the cost of treatment for specific patients.

Control measures Ways in which risk can be controlled, including physical controls such as locking away drugs and valuable items, and system controls such as restricting access to hazardous areas to specific staff groups.

Convenor A non-executive director of a trust, health authority or health board who decides whether or not to convene an independent panel to review a complaint against an NHS provider.

Corporate Relating to the whole of an organisation, e.g. the management of an organisation.

Corporate seal A seal used by organisations to certify documents used in legal transactions (such as the sale of land) so as to fulfil legal requirements.

Court welfare officer (children) Officer appointed to provide a report for the court about the child and the child's family situation and background. The court welfare officer will usually be a probation officer.

Criterion A measurable component of performance. A number of criteria need to be met to achieve the desired standard.

Cross-functional team A team of people from different disciplines.

Cruse A non-religious UK-based organisation specialising in bereavement. Email info@crusebereavementcare.org.uk

Cybernetics A name coined by Norbert Weiner in the 1950s to describe the study of feedback control systems and their application. Such systems were seen to exhibit properties associated with human intelligence and robotics, and so were an early contribution to the theory of artificial intelligence.

Cyberspace Popular term (now associated with the Internet) which describes the notional information 'space' that is created across computer networks. (*See also* virtual reality.)

Cycle time Time a patient is under treatment (in hospital). Thus, cycle time plus waiting time equals the lead time.

Database A structured repository for data, usually stored on a computer system. The existence of a regular and formal indexing structure permits rapid retrieval of individual elements of the database.

Day care (children) A person provides day care if they look after one or more children under the age of eight on non-domestic premises for more than two hours in any day.

Day cases   Patients who have an investigation, treatment or operation, but are admitted electively and discharged on the same day.

Decision support system   General term for any computer application that enhances a human's ability to make decisions.

Decision tree   A method of representing knowledge that makes structured decisions in a hierarchical tree-like fashion.

Deduction   A method of logical inference. Given a cause, deduction infers all logical effects that might arise as a consequence. (*See also* abduction, induction and inference.)

Designated person   A person within an NHS provider, or a department of an NHS provider, who is delegated responsibility to ensure that complaints are properly resolved locally.

Detailed records   At present patients have many detailed records. These include a GP record, usually held electronically but often supplemented by paper records. Where patients have visited a hospital or clinic, there will usually be an electronic patient administration record; a separate written clinical record in their local hospital; a separate paper record if they have been pregnant; a further separate paper record if they have received mental health treatment; another separate paper record if they have been treated in the sexual health clinic; and a separate record if they have attended Accident and Emergency. Each of these records will be repeated for each hospital or clinic the patient has attended. In addition, the patient may have a community record if receiving long-term care in the community (e.g. physiotherapy). The National Programme for IT has a clear objective to reduce this duplication of diverse records by providing a patient-centred electronic detailed record that spans these areas. As a minimum, this would be within a hospital but there are real benefits when providing a consistent record across a local health community and across the boundaries involved in care pathways for a patient. The overall objective is a single detailed record for an individual patient that is accessible by the GP and by community and local hospital care settings.

Dictionary of Medicines and Devices (dm+d)   The source of terminology and a common language for medicines and devices used in healthcare.

Direct credits   The income from the sale of meals to staff, renting accommodation to staff and so on.

Direct discrimination   Where someone is treated less favourably purely on grounds of marital status, sex, ethnic origin or similar criteria which do not affect the individual's ability to perform the job. (*See also* indirect discrimination)

Disabled (children)   A child is disabled if 'he or she is blind, deaf or dumb or suffers from a mental disorder of any kind or is substantially and permanently handicapped by illness, injury or congenital deformity or such other disability'.

Dissent to share   *See* consent to share.

Disclosure interview (children)   Term sometimes used to indicate an interview with a child, conducted as part of the assessment for suspected sexual abuse. It could be misleading (since it implies, in some people's view, undue pressure on the child to 'disclose') and therefore the latest preferred term is 'investigative interview'.

Discrimination   May be direct or indirect. For details see separate headings.

Distributed computing   Term for computer systems in which data and programs are distributed and shared across different computers on a network.

Dual registered homes   Homes for disabled or elderly people, registered as both a residential care home and a nursing home.

Duty to investigate (children)   A local authority is under a duty to investigate in a number of situations where they have a 'reasonable cause to suspect that a child who lives, or is found, in [its] area is suffering, or is likely to suffer, significant harm'.

Early Adopter Programme   A programme of work involving NHS Connecting for Health supporting the first primary care trusts to implement Summary Care Records for patients in their area. There were six Early Adopter PCTs that made up the Early Adopter Programme. The Early Adopter sites were independently evaluated so that lessons could be learned and business processes tested and refined before Summary Care Records started to roll out across England from 2008.

European Computer Driving Licence (ECDL)   A training course in essential IT skills available to all NHS staff to help them prepare for new ways of working and increase confidence in their use of IT. ECDL is an internationally recognised qualification that has been adopted as the NHS standard. Since replaced by Essential IT Skills.

Education supervision order (children)   Order which puts a child under the supervision of a designated local education authority.

Education welfare officer (EWO)   Social work support to children in the context of their schooling. While EWOs' main focus used to be the enforcement of school attendance, today they perform a wider range of services, including seeking to ensure that children receive adequate and appropriate education and that any special needs are met, and more general liaison between local authority education and social services departments.

Educational psychologist A psychology graduate who has had teaching experience and additional vocational training. Educational psychologists perform a range of functions including assessing children's education, psychological and emotional needs, offering therapy and contributing psychological expertise to the process of assessment.

Electronic mail *See* email.

Electronic medical record A general term describing computer-based patient record systems. It is sometimes extended to include other functions, such as order entry for medications and tests, among other common functions.

electronic Government Interoperability Framework (eGIF) Standards used to ensure the security of systems for registering system users and authenticating their identity. The eGIF defines the technical policies and specifications governing information flows across government and the public sector.

Electronic Patient Record (EPR) EPR is a catch-all term covering the patient data held in digital form by computers. The National Programme for IT is delivering a number of EPRs. A Summary Care Record (SCR), Detailed Records, Diagnostic Test Order and Results, PACS images and all other clinical data held in computers are examples of EPRs.

Electronic transmission of prescriptions (ETP) Enables GPs/prescribers to send prescriptions electronically to pharmacies.

Email/e-mail/electronic mail A messaging system available on computer networks, providing users with personal mail boxes from which electronic messages can be sent and received.

Emergency admission A patient admitted on the same day that admission is requested.

Emergency protection order (children) That which a court can make if it is satisfied that a child is likely to suffer significant harm, or where inquiries are being made with respect to the child and they are being frustrated by the unreasonable refusal of access to the child.

End of life Patients are 'approaching the end of life' when they are likely to die within the next 12 months. This category includes those where death is expected within hours or days; those who have advanced, progressive incurable conditions; those with general frailty and co-existing conditions that mean they are expected to die within 12 months; those at risk of dying from a sudden acute crisis in an existing condition; and those with life-threatening acute conditions caused by sudden catastrophic events. The term can also be applied to extremely premature neonates whose prospects for survival are known to be very poor and patients who are diagnosed as being in a persistent vegetative state for whom a decision to withdraw treatment and care may lead to their death.

End stage   The final period in the course of a progressive disease leading to a patient's death.

Enterprise-wide arrangements   Arrangements with key suppliers in the IT industry. Given its size, the National Programme seeks to procure quality IT services from suppliers to the NHS on a greater scale and at a more competitive rate than any single NHS organisation.

Epidemiology   Study of the distribution and determinants of disease in human populations.

Epistemology   The philosophical study of knowledge.

Estates strategy   A written statement of objectives relating to estates management and a plan for meeting those objectives. The strategy should be consistent with the business plan.

European Directive   A requirement which binds an EU member state, e.g. the one designed to facilitate the free movement of doctors and the mutual recognition of their diplomas, certificates and other evidence of formal qualifications (Council Directive 93/16/EEC).

Evaluation   The study of the performance of a service (or element of treatment and care) with the aim of identifying successful and problem areas of activity.

Evidence-based medicine   A movement advocating the practice of medicine according to clinical guidelines, developed to reflect best practice as captured from a meta-analysis of the clinical literature. (*See also* clinical guideline, meta-analysis and protocol.)

Existing system provider   A supplier whose system is currently installed within the NHS and related care settings. NHS Connecting for Health's Existing Systems Programme works with these suppliers to make their systems compatible with National Programme systems and services that in turn ought to enable patients to benefit from the new services such as Choose and Book, the Electronic Prescription Service and GP2GP Record Transfer.

Expert system A computer program that contains expert knowledge about a particular problem, often in the form of a set of if-then rules, that is able to solve problems at a level equivalent or greater than human experts. (*See also* artificial intelligence.)

Explicit consent *See* consent to share.

External financing limit (EFL) A cash limit set by the NHSE on net external financing for an NHS trust. A positive external financing limit is set where the agreed capital spending for an NHS trust exceeds income from internally generated resources. A zero external financing limit is set where the agreed capital spending programme for a trust equals internally generated resources. A negative external financing limit is set where the agreed capital spending programme for a trust is less than internally generated resources.

Extra-contractual referral (ECR) The term used for referral of an individual for health services that were not covered in contracts that existed between the old system of purchaser and providers of services.

Family centre Child and parents, or other person looking after a child, can attend for occupational and recreational activities, advice, guidance or counselling, and accommodation while receiving such advice, guidance or counselling.

Family Panel Panel from which magistrates who sit in the new Family Proceedings Court are selected. These magistrates will have undergone specialist training on the Children's Act.

Family Proceedings Court Court at the level of the magistrates' court to hear proceedings under the Children Act 1989. The magistrates will be selected from a new panel, known as the Family Panel, and will be specially trained.

Fieldworker (field social worker) Conducts a range of social work functions in the community and in other settings (e.g. hospitals).

Financial strategy A written statement of objectives relating to financial management and a plan for meeting those objectives. The strategy should be consistent with the business plan.

Financial target (for an NHS trust) A real pre-interest return of 6% on the value of net assets, effectively a return on the average of the opening and closing assets shown in the accounts.

Finished consultant episode (FCE) An episode where the patient has completed a period of care under a consultant and is either discharged or transferred to another consultant. The total number of episodes is a common measure of overall hospital activity.

Firewall   A security barrier erected between a public computer network like the Internet and a local private computer network.

Flexible training   Available for doctors who have 'well-founded individual reasons' for working less than full-time. The DoH runs two schemes to encourage flexible training for career registrars and senior registrars (PM(79)3). Flexible training for PRHOs and SHOs is available on a personal basis. In addition, a number of regions organise their own flexible training schemes.

Foster carer   Provides substitute family care for children. A child looked after by a local authority can be placed with local authority foster carers.

Foundation trusts (FTs)   First set up as a result of the Health and Social Care (Community Health and Standards) Act 2003. More hospitals have become foundation trusts since then and all Acute NHS Trusts will be required to attain FT status by the end of 2008. Although remaining part of the NHS, foundation trusts are subject to reduced control from central government. They differ from traditional NHS trusts in three main ways:

▶ they possess the freedom to decide locally how to meet their obligations (which can also involve borrowing money from private sources)

▶ they are accountable, through (mainly elected) governors, to their members, who are drawn from local residents, patients and staff

▶ they are authorised and monitored by Monitor, the Independent Regulator of NHS foundation trusts.

Frequently asked questions (FAQ)   Common term for information lists available on the Internet which have been compiled for newcomers on a particular subject, answering common questions that would otherwise often be asked by submitting email requests to a Newsgroup.

Front line staff   The employees of an NHS provider who have direct, face-to-face contact with patients and other NHS users.

Front Line Support Academy   Provides learning opportunities for staff involved in the implementation of IT in the NHS and social care. The Academy works with staff to change and improve patients' experience of their care.

Functional department   Examples would include X-ray, a ward, theatre, pharmacy, pathology, a clinic or outpatients.

Functional team   A team from within a single discipline.

General Practice Element   Usually referenced in relation to Summary

Care Records, this is the information from the GP patient record that is included in a patient's Summary Care Record.

General Medical Services (GMS)   The rules used to manage payments to family doctors as part of the GP's contract.

General Medical Services Contract (GMS contract)   In 2003 GPs accepted a new contract, negotiated by the British Medical Association and the NHS Confederation. The terms of this contract meant that payments to GPs were more closely related to the quantity and quality of the services provided.

Go live   For the purposes of communications with the public, go live is when new systems and services start to be used to enable information to be linked so that it can be accessed by people in different organisations, e.g. a hospital can access information created by a GP.

GP fundholder   Term that was used for GP practice with a budget for the purchase of a range of hospital inpatient and outpatient (and certain nursing and paramedical) services. Ceased in April 1999.

GP2GP   A service that transfers electronic patient records from one GP practice to another when a patient changes GP practices. A secure way of transferring patient records from one GP practice to another.

Guardian *ad litem* (GAL)   Person appointed by a court to investigate a child's circumstances and to report to the court.

Guidance (children)   Authorities are required to act in accordance with the guidance issued by the Secretary of State. However, guidance does not have the full force of law but is intended as a series of statements of good practice and may be quoted or used in court proceedings.

Hawthorne effect   Term used to describe changes in productivity and employee morale as a direct result of management interest in their problems. Improvements may arise before any management action. Originates from a study of the Hawthorne Works, Western Electric Co, USA (1920s).

Hazard assessment procedures   The process by which the origins, frequencies, costs and effects of hazards are identified and strategies adopted to avoid or minimise their effects.

Hazards   The potential to cause harm, including ill health and injury, damage to property, plant, products or the environment, production losses or increased liabilities.

Health and safety policy   A plan of action for the health, safety and well-being of staff, patients, residents and visitors.

Healthcare Resource Groups (HRGs)   These are codes that signify clinically similar treatments that use common levels of healthcare resource. An information management tool, they have been developed to support Payment by Results.

Health economy or health community   These terms generally refer to all providers, purchasers and service users within a defined geographical area.

Health gain   The improvement of the health status of a community or population. It is sometimes described as 'adding years to life and life to years'.

Health level 7 (HL7)   A healthcare-specific communication standard for data exchange between computer applications.

Healthcare professional   A person qualified in a health discipline.

Health promotion   Enabling individuals and communities to increase control over the determinants of health and thereby improve their health.

Health record   Information about the physical or mental health of someone, which has been made by, or on behalf of, a health professional in connection with the care of that person. These must be kept for a statutory period of time after the patient is discharged from the service. Records will be held in addition to care plans.

Health Service Commissioner (HSC)   The Ombudsman, appointed by Parliament to protect the rights of users of the NHS. Responsible only to Parliament.

Health service price index   This index takes the NHS 'shopping basket' of goods and services (it excludes pay of employees) and weighs them according to use. The cost movement of these items is measured each month and the index updated to reflect these changes. It is used by the NHS to measure price movements and quite often to update allocations and budgets.

HealthSpace   A secure website which provides an online personal health organiser for patients. In time, and after completing the registration process for an advanced HealthSpace account, patients who have a Summary Care Record will be able to access it using HealthSpace.

Health status   A measure of the overall health experience of an individual or a defined population.

Hearing   The process of perceiving sound or agreement to having heard a person's statement.

Herzberg's two-factor theory   Herzberg maintained on the basis of research studies that in any work there are factors which satisfy and dissatisfy, but they are not necessarily opposites of each other. The latter are to do with conditions of work which he called hygiene or maintenance factors, and the former are achievement, recognition, responsibility and advancement, which he called motivators.

Heuristic A rule of thumb that describes how things are commonly understood, without resorting to deeper or more formal knowledge. (*See also* model-based reasoning.)

HMRL First of a series of hospital medical record forms. It is usually the front sheet of a patient's case notes and summarises personal, administrative and medical details. It is used for inpatients in all hospitals except those for mental illness and maternity.

Hospice NHS, voluntary or private residential premises for the provision of clinical and nursing care to residents who are terminally ill.

Hospital acquired infection An infection acquired by a patient during their stay in hospital, which is unconnected with their reason for admission.

Hospital information system (HIS) Typically used to describe hospital computer systems with functions such as patient admission and discharge, order entry for laboratory tests or medications, and billing functions. (*See also* electronic medical record.)

Hospital stay The number of days a patient stays on one hospital site during a hospital provider spell.

Hotel costs The costs of food, heating, maintenance and so on for keeping a patient in hospital, excluding all medical and treatment costs.

Human-computer interaction The study of the psychology and design principles associated with the way humans interact with computer systems.

Human-computer interface The 'view' presented by a program to its user. Often literally a visual window that allows a program to be operated, an interface could just as easily be based on the recognition and synthesis of speech or any other medium with which a human is able to sense or manipulate.

Human resource strategy A written statement of human resource objectives and a plan for meeting those objectives. The strategy should be consistent with the business plan.

Hygiene factor The element of work motivation concerned with the environment or context of job, i.e. salary, status and security, etc. To be distinguished from motivators, i.e. achievement recognition. Based on theory of Herzberg F. (*see* Herzberg 1959).

IG alert   An alert to a Caldicott Guardian or Privacy Officer, which will be generated when a user has had to justify special access to confidential patient information, and access has been provided. The privacy officer will ensure that the reason given for access is genuine and justifiable.

Information Governance (IG)   The structures, policies and practice used to ensure the confidentiality and security of health and social care services records, especially clinical records, and to enable the ethical use of them for the benefit of the individual to whom they relate and for the public good.

IG Statement of Compliance (IGSoC)   An agreement between NHS Connecting for Health and any organisation wishing to use services provided through the National Programme for IT. The agreement stipulates the obligations that the organisation is expected to maintain to ensure patient data is safeguarded and only used appropriately.

Implied consent   *See* consent to share.

In care (children)   Refers to a child in the care of the local authority by virtue of an order or under an interim order.

Incident   An event or occurrence, especially one that leads to problems. An example of this could be an attack on one person by another within a service.

Income and expenditure reports   An accountancy tool which describes and analyses the flow of funds into and out of an organisation in order to assess liquidity. Sometimes known as 'source and application of funds statements' or more commonly 'cash flow statements'.

Independent contractor   In primary care, this normally refers to a self-employed professional. The vast majority of GPs are self-employed – unlike hospital doctors who are normally directly employed by the hospital.

Independent review   The process of a panel of laypersons reviewing the case of a complaint where the complainant is not satisfied with the results of local resolution by an NHS provider.

Independent visitor (children)   A local authority in certain sets of circumstances appoints such a visitor for a child it is looking after. The visitor appointed has the duty of 'visiting, advising and befriending the child'.

Indirect discrimination   Where an unjustifiable requirement or condition is applied to the job which has a disproportionately adverse effect on one sex or group. For example, the career and life pattern of women is often different from that of men as a consequence of family responsibilities and child-bearing. Women may be less mobile than men. Another example of indirect discrimination is insisting on a conventional career path. (*See also* direct discrimination.)

Individual performance review (IPR) A system of appraisal based on the setting of agreed objectives and targets between individual employees and their managers and the extent of the attainment of these targets. Normally, IPR is linked to development; within the NHS it is often associated with performance-related pay for senior managers.

Induction A method of logical inference used to suggest relationships from observations. This is the process of generalisation we use to create models of the world. (*See also* abduction, deduction and inference.)

Induction programme Learning activities designed to enable newly appointed staff to function effectively in a new position.

Industrial tribunals Set up under the Industrial Training Act 1964, they consider cases of unfair dismissal, sex discrimination and disability.

Industry Liaison Provides information and guidance to IT suppliers who would like to be involved in providing products and services to NPfIT. It also supplies information to the National Programme on product innovations and developments in IT.

Infant mortality rate The deaths of infants under one year of age per 1000 live births.

Inference A logical conclusion drawn using one of several methods of reasoning, knowledge and data. (*See also* abduction, deduction and induction.)

Information Governance Framework The Information Governance Framework for Health and Social Care is formed by those elements of law and policy from which applicable information governance standards are derived, and the activities and roles which individually and collectively ensure that these standards are clearly defined and met. While a key focus of information governance is the use of information about service users, it applies to information and information processing in its broadest sense and underpins both clinical and corporate governance.

Information Standards Board (ISB) Established in 2001 to provide an independent mechanism for the approval of information standards in the NHS.

Information superhighway A popular term associated with the Internet and used to describe its role in the global mass transportation of information.

Information theory Initially developed by Claude Shannon, this describes the amount of data that can be transmitted across a channel given specific encoding techniques and noise in the signal.

Informed consent The legal principle by which a patient is informed about the nature, purpose and likely effects of any treatment proposed, before being asked to consent to accepting it.

Inherent jurisdiction (children) Powers of High Court to make orders to protect a child.

Injunction Order made by the court prohibiting an act or requiring its cessation.

Inpatient A patient who has gone through the full admission procedure and is occupying a bed in a hospital inpatients' department.

Inquisitorial One of two kinds of court process: adversarial and inquisitorial. The inquisitorial system is one where the role of the court is to inquire into the facts of a particular matter in order to reach a judgement. The Coroners Court is a good example.

Inspiration trap The difficulty faced by a conciliator who can identify an obvious and sensible solution to a dispute but must ensure that the parties to the dispute reach the same conclusion without identifiable direction from the conciliator.

Integrated Services Digital Network (ISDN) A digital telephone network that is designed to provide channels for voice and data services. Customer must be within about 3.4 miles of the telephone exchange otherwise expensive repeater devices are required.

Inter-agency plan (children) Plan devised jointly by the agencies concerned in a child's welfare which co-ordinates the services they provide.

Interim Access Controls All NHS organisations are working towards fulfilling all the commitments set out in the Care Record Guarantee. Until that time, interim measures will be put in place by organisations, in order to allow appropriate access to information while providing the necessary security and confidentiality.

Interim care order (children) Made by court, placing the child in the care of the designated local authority.

International Classification of Disease (ICD-10) Tenth edition published by the World Health Organization for the statistical classification of morbidity and mortality. It may be used in conjunction with another classification termed Read coding. Review of the

WHO website suggests work is under way on ICD-11 and more information about the ICD can be found at www.who.int/research/en.

Investigative interview (children) Preferred term for an interview conducted with a child as part of an assessment following concerns that the child may have been abused.

Investment appraisal A means of assessing whether expenditure of capital (or revenue) on a project will show a satisfactory rate of return (e.g. lower costs or higher income), either absolutely or when compared with alternative projects.

Job description Contains standard information for staff regarding conditions of service, location(s) of the post, duties of the post, accountability, education and training facilities, appraisal and the salary scale of the post. It should be available and made known to all potential applicants at the earliest possible stage and should be sent out with every application form. It contains details of accountability, responsibility, formal lines of communication, principal duties, entitlements and performance review. It is a guide for an individual in a specific position within an organisation. (*See also* person specification.)

Joint financing A sum of money taken from the health allocation and then spent on projects which are agreed by a joint consultative committee. Such monies should normally be spent on personal social service projects to reduce demands on NHS services.

Judicial review An order from the divisional court quashing a disputed decision. The divisional court cannot substitute its own decision but can merely send the matter back to the offending authority for reconsideration.

Key worker The person responsible for co-ordinating the care plan for each individual patient, for monitoring its progress and for staying in regular contact with the patient and everyone involved. A key worker may be from a variety of different professional or non-professional backgrounds.

Kipling's serving men 'I keep six honest serving men (they taught me all I know). Their names are What and Why and When and How and Where and Who'.

Knowledge acquisition Subspecialty of artificial intelligence, usually associated with developing methods for capturing human knowledge and of converting it into a form that can be used by computer. (*See also* expert system, heuristic and machine learning.)

Knowledge-based system *See* expert system.

Korner data Korner relates to the review of NHS information requirements by the NHS/DHSS steering group on health services information which was chaired by Edith Korner. The group recommended a minimum set of data that should be collected in all districts for management purposes.

Lay person A person who is not, and preferably never has been, a professional in the field under dispute or any associated field.

Lead time Time between presentation to GP or perhaps A&E and discharge. Thus the lead time = cycle time + waiting time.

Lecture 50–55 minutes of largely uninterrupted discourse from a teacher with no discussion between students and no student activity other than listening and note taking.

Legacy systems suppliers These are the commercial companies that supply the current/existing IT systems and software in use in the NHS. Also known as existing systems suppliers.

Legal proxy Person with legal authority to make decisions on behalf of another adult. Legal proxies who can make healthcare decisions include: a person holding a lasting Power of Attorney (England and Wales) or a Welfare Power of Attorney (Scotland); a court appointed deputy (England and Wales); and a court appointed guardian or court appointed intervener (Scotland). Northern Ireland currently has no provision for appointing legal proxies with the power to make healthcare decisions.

Legitimate relationship (LR) Staff involved in a patient's care are considered to have a 'legitimate relationship' with that patient. Access to confidential information will be limited to those staff who have a 'legitimate relationship' with that patient.

Listen The process of actively hearing, accepting and understanding a verbal communication.

Local Improvement Finance Trust (LIFT) Local Improvement Finance Trusts are a method for funding primary care and community care estates modernisation, similar in some respects to PFI. The contracts involved in a LIFT scheme are for buildings and maintenance. It is an additional procurement route for developing primary care estates that currently includes the use of conventional public capital, premises built and operated under the national contract for general medical services (GMS), PFI and other public–private partnerships.

Local implementation An NPfIT management group and individual project teams who have responsibilities for implementation in each SHA. They co-ordinate and manage the progress of the programme by dealing with a variety of issues, including progress monitoring, problem solving, risk management, planning, good practice and allocating resources.

Local resolution The process of resolving a complaint against an NHS provider swiftly, at or very near to the point at which the issue complained about actually occurred.

Local Service Providers (LSPs) Responsible for working with the local NHS to deliver National Programme for IT systems and services at a local level. They work to integrate local systems with national applications and to maintain common standards. LSPs also support local organisations to deliver and realise the benefits from their National Programme for IT systems and services.

Local voices initiative Encourages gathering of the views and wishes of local people as a contribution to purchasing intelligence (q.v.).

Logical To follow a sound set of rules and tests.

Looked after (children) A child is looked after when in local authority care or is being provided with accommodation by the local authority.

Mailing list A list of email addresses for individuals. Used to distribute information to small groups of individuals who may, for example, have shared interests. (*See also* email.)

Major incident (external) A serious external incident which requires the organisation to implement contingency plans or change or suspend some normal functions. An example would be the aftermath of a rail crash.

Major incident (internal) A serious incident occurring within the healthcare facility resulting in the changing or suspension of some normal functions or threatening of the organisation. This requires the drawing up of contingency plans. Examples of this would include the loss of electricity or telecommunications services or bomb threats.

Makaton symbols A system of symbols used to communicate with some people who have severe learning disabilities.

Management by objectives An approach to management which aims to integrate the organisation's objectives with the individual's objectives.

Management development An approach for ensuring that the organisation meets its current and future needs for effective managers. Would include succession planning, performance appraisal and training.

Manpower planning   A method of ensuring that the organisation's human resources can be met now and in the future.

Market forces   May be characterised as any system of incentives which rely on market type mechanisms such as contracts, price or cost to create a desired behaviour from the various participants in that market. For example, competition, fixed or decreasing budget limits, bidding for contracts, and so on may all be seen as market forces.

Matrix management   A system of managing in a horizontal as well as a vertical organisation structure. Typically, a person reports to two superiors, a department or line manager and a functional or project manager.

Matrix team   People from different parts of the organisation and with no line authority.

Mediation   The process of resolving a dispute by the intervention of an expert person who closely guides the disputing parties towards agreement.

Mentoring and co-mentoring   An ancient process of learning facilitation by mutual professional support, traditionally given by a senior to a junior colleague. In co-mentoring the process of mentoring is non-hierarchical and involves co-mentees helping and supporting each other in learning.

Meta-analysis   Pooled statistical analysis of results from several individual statistical analyses of different experiments, searching for statistical significance which is not possible within the smaller sample sizes of individual studies.

Mind map   A process of recording information in related groupings which is intended to assist lateral thinking. (*See also* cognitive map.)

Minimum data sets   A group of statistics or other information that together comprise the minimum amount of information required to inform any management process, for example for contract monitoring.

Ministerial Taskforce   An NHS Summary Care Record Taskforce was established in July 2006 to recommend how best to implement the Summary Care Record in the Early Adopter Programme. It reported to ministers in December 2006 and its recommendations are being implemented. The Taskforce considered a variety of perspectives including clinicians, hospital managers, patients and the ambulance service.

Mission statement   Statement of the overall purpose of an organisation.

Model Any representation of a real object or phenomenon, or template for the creation of an object or phenomenon.

Model-based reasoning Approach to the development of expert systems that uses formally defined models of systems, in contrast to more superficial rules of thumbs. (*See also* artificial intelligence and heuristic.)

Modernisation Agency Created as part of the NHS Plan to help local clinicians and managers redesign local services around the needs and convenience of patients. It is discussed in more detail in Chapter 1, 'Understanding the NHS' of *A Guide to the NHS*.

Monitor An independent corporate body established under the Health and Social Care (Community Health and Standards) Act 2003. It is responsible for authorising, monitoring and regulating NHS foundation trusts.

Monitoring The systematic process of collecting information on clinical and non-clinical performance. Monitoring may be intermittent or continuous. It may also be undertaken in relation to specific incidents of concern or to check key performance areas. It is also used in respect of selection in recording data such as sex, ethnic origin and age, etc. on applicants, short-listed candidates and appointees for retrospective review to show whether an organisation's equal opportunities policies are being carried out successfully. Monitoring also includes analysing the information and data obtained to see if there are any discrepancies in treatment/success rates of different groups, identifying the reasons and taking remedial action where appropriate. Monitoring in respect of childcare is where plans for a child, and the child's safety and well-being, are systematically appraised on a routine basis. Its function is to oversee the child's continued welfare and enable any necessary action or change to be instigated speedily, and, at a managerial level, to ensure that proper professional standards are being maintained.

Morbidity The incidence of a particular disease or group of diseases in a given population during a specified period of time.

Mortality The number of deaths in a given population during a specified period of time.

Motivators Factors leading to job satisfaction and high employee morale. *See* Herzberg's theory of motivation, as described in some detail on p. 118 in *The Doctor's Handbook, Part 1*. Also *see* Herzberg 1983.

Movement The stage in a conciliation or mediation process during which the parties modify their views and their opinions become closer to each other's.

Multi-professional A combination of several professions working towards a common aim.

National Application Service Providers (NASPs) Responsible for purchasing and integrating IT systems and services which are common to all users across the country including the Spine element of the NHS Care Records Service, Choose and Book, NHSmail and the National Network for the NHS (N3).

National clinical leads Appointed by NHS Connecting for Health to lead engagement about the National Programme for IT with their respective clinical professions at a national level. National clinical leads are in place for nurses, GPs and hospital doctors. They work closely with the clinical professional bodies and other organisations as well as the chief clinical officers at the DoH. They make sure that clinical involvement is central to all the work of NHS Connecting for Health.

National Programme for IT (NPfIT) Responsible for procurement and delivery of the multi-billion-pound investment in new information and technology systems to improve the NHS.

National Information Governance Board for Health and Social Care Provides leadership and promotes consistent standards for information governance across health and social care. It arbitrates on the interpretation and application of information governance policy and gives advice on matters at national level. The NIGB has taken over some of the responsibilities of the Care Record Development Board, which has now closed. It will continue to publish and review the NHS Care Record Guarantee.

National Network for the NHS (N3) Provides fast, wide area networking services to the NHS, offering reliability and value for money. N3 replaced the private NHS communications network NHSnet. N3 is vital to the delivery of the National Programme for IT, providing the essential technical infrastructure to support the NHS Care Records Service, the Electronic Prescription Service, Choose and Book and Picture Archiving and Communications Systems.

National Service Frameworks (NSFs) Set national standards and service models for a specific service or care group. They set up programmes of implementation and performance management against which progress in an agreed timescale can be measured. They may help decide which services are best provided in primary care, in hospitals and in specialist centres.

Natural team   For example, a boss with direct subordinates.

Neonatal death rate   The deaths of infants under four weeks of age per 1000 live births. The early neonatal death rate is the deaths of infants under one week of age per 1000 live births.

Neonates   Newborn infants less than one month old.

Neural computing   *See* connectionism.

Neural network   Computer program or system designed to mimic some aspects of neurone connections, including summation of action potentials, refractory periods and firing thresholds.

New outpatient   A patient attending for an outpatient appointment for the first time for a particular ailment. If transferred to another department, the patient is also a new outpatient on their first attendance there.

Newsgroup   A bulletin board service provided on a computer network like the Internet, where messages can be sent by email and be viewed by those who have an interest in the contents of a particular newsgroup. (*See also* email and Internet.)

NHS Care Records Service (NHS CRS)   A secure service that links patient information from different parts of the NHS electronically so authorised NHS staff and patients have the information they need to make care decisions. There are two elements to the NHS CRS: detailed records (held locally) and the Summary Care Record (held nationally). The NHS CRS enables each person's detailed records to be securely shared between different parts of the local NHS, such as the GP surgery and hospital. Patients will also be able to have a summary of their important health information, known as their Summary Care Record, available to authorised NHS staff treating them anywhere in the NHS in England. Patients will be able to access their Summary Care Record using the secure website HealthSpace.

NHS Code of Practice   Sets out the basic principles underlying public access to information about the NHS. It reflects the government's intention to ensure greater access by the public to information about public services and complements the Code of Access to Information which applies to the DoH.

NHS Connecting for Health (NHS CFH)   An agency of the DoH supporting the NHS to introduce the National Programme for IT. This will help the NHS to deliver better, safer care for patients. NHS CFH is also responsible for other existing business-critical IT systems in the NHS.

NHSmail   A secure national email and directory service. It was developed specifically to meet NHS and BMA requirements for clinical email between NHS organisations.

NHS Number The NHS Number is fundamental to the National Programme for IT. It is the national unique patient identifier that makes it possible to share patient information across the whole of the NHS safely, efficiently and accurately.

NHS Plan Recognises that the NHS has achieved much but needs to keep pace with change to meet patient needs. Increased investment and modernisation are the steps described in the document (it was published July 2000).

Non-principals A generic term for doctors who wish to practise in general practice but who do not want the financial or time commitment of becoming a principal – includes retainers, returners, assistants and associates as well as the new salaried doctor opportunities available under Primary Care Act Pilots (PCAPs).

Non-recurrent expenditure 'One-off expenditure', e.g. provision of new buildings, major alterations and major pieces of equipment. Clearly, capital expenditure is non-recurrent expenditure but the purchase of minor pieces of equipment and the carrying out of maintenance work is non-recurrent, though chargeable to revenue.

Non-recurring measures These are one-off measures which affect the year of account only, e.g. raising capital through the sale of land or via a one-off payment or loan from an external source such as the Strategic Health Authority NHS Bank.

Objective A clearly identifiable and quantifiable target to be achieved in the future. A specific and measurable statement which also sets out how overall aims are to be achieved.

Office of Population, Census and Surveys (OPCS) The central government office that collected information on the entire population. Now Office for National Statistics.

Official solicitor Officer of the Supreme Court. When representing a child, the official solicitor acts as a solicitor as well as a guardian *ad litem*.

Ombudsman Health Service Commissioner who investigates cases of maladministration in the health service.

Open-loop control Partially automated control method in which a part of the control system is given over to humans.

Open system Computer industry term for computer hardware and software that is built to common public standards, allowing purchasers to select components from a variety of vendors and to use them together.

Opinion   A belief which is held but may not be based on provable fact.

Organisation   A generic term used to describe an entire organisation, as opposed to the term service, which is used to describe one part of the organisation (*see also* service). Thus a hospital, a practice or a university or medical school may all be described as organisations.

Organisation and management development strategy   A written document which sets out the strategy for developing the organisational processes and management skills needed by an organisation.

Organisational chart   A graphical representation of the structure of the organisation, including areas of responsibility, relationships and formal lines of communication and accountability.

Organisational development (OD)   An educational strategy aimed at changing the beliefs, attitudes, values and structures within an organisation so that it can better adapt to changing requirements. The emphasis is on interventions, rather than the objective assessment of services. A systematic process of improving organisational effectiveness and adaptiveness on the basis of behavioural science knowledge.

Originating capital debt   The amount owed by an NHS trust to the consolidated fund. This is equal to the value of the net assets transferred to an NHS trust when it is set up. Assets donated to the NHS since 1948 are not included.

Output-based specification (OBS)   Each prospective supplier to the National Programme must meet rigorous technical requirements. These are set out in an output-based specification.

Outcome   The effect on health status of a healthcare intervention or lack of intervention. The end result of care and treatment; that is, the change in health, functional ability, symptoms or situation of a person, which can be used to measure the effectiveness of care and treatment.

Outpatient   A patient attending for treatment, consultation, advice and so on, but not staying in a hospital.

Output (or programme) budgets   A system of analysing expenditure by reference to objectives to be met (e.g. increased level of day care; more operations) instead of under input headings such as staff and running expenses, etc.

Out-turn prices   The prices prevailing when the expenditure occurs, as distinct from the estimated prices.

Overall benefit   The ethical basis on which decisions are made about treatment and care for adult patients who lack a capacity to decide for themselves. This involves appropriateness of treatment not only the potential clinical benefits, burdens and risks but non-clinical factors such as the patient's personal circumstances, wishes, beliefs and values. There is GMC guidance on this consistent with the legal requirement to consider whether treatment is in the patient's 'best interests' (England, Wales and Northern Ireland), or 'benefits' a patient (Scotland). It also takes into account other principles set out in the Mental Capacity Act 2005 and the Adults with Incapacity (Scotland) Act 2000.

Palliative care   The holistic care of patients with advanced, progressive or incurable illness focused on the management of a patient's pain and other distressing symptoms and the provision of psychological, social and spiritual support to patients and their family. Palliative care is not dependent on diagnosis or prognosis and can be provided at any stage of a patient's illness not only in the last few days of life. The objective is to support patients to live as well as possible until they die and to die with dignity.

Paramedics   Ambulance personnel with extended qualifications in providing pre-hospital care according to protocols.

Paramount principle   The principle that the welfare of the child is the paramount consideration in proceedings concerning children.

Parental responsibility   Defined as all the rights, duties, powers, responsibilities and authority which by law a parent of a child has in relation to the child and his property.

Part III accommodation   Residential care homes provided by local authorities under Part III of the National Assistance Act 1948.

Parties   Parties to legal proceedings under the Children's Act are entitled to attend the hearing, present their case and examine witnesses. The Act envisages that children will automatically be parties in care proceedings. Anyone with parental responsibility for the child will also be a party to such proceedings, as will the local authority. Others may be able to acquire party status.

Party   A patient, carer, representative or NHS provider involved in a dispute.

Passcode   An alphanumeric code unique to each member of NHS staff to use alongside their Smartcard to access patient information contained on the patient's care record.

Patient   A person currently or previously under medical care.

Patient Advice and Liaison Service (PALS)   Known as PALS, the Patient Advice and Liaison Service supports patients to ensure that the NHS listens to patients, their relatives, carers and friends; answers their questions and resolves their concerns as quickly as possible.

PALS also helps the NHS to improve services by listening to what matters to patients and their carers and supporting the NHS to make changes, when appropriate.

Patient Administration System (PAS) An administrative system typically used in hospitals and community service settings that contain essential non-clinical data, such as patient attendance lists, appointments and waiting times.

Patient and Public Involvement Forums (PPI Forums) PPI Forums were set up following the NHS Reform and Health Care Professions Act 2002. There are 572 forums – one for each trust in England. They are the local voice of the community on health matters and have a wide range of responsibilities.

Patient costing A system whereby costs are analysed in relation to specific patients or types of patient. This is the most complete analysis that can be undertaken and enables different combinations of costs to be made to fulfil any requirement. Particularly useful for evaluating proposed changes in service provision.

The Patient's Charter A list of required national standards and rights set by central government for the NHS.

Patients' council/forum/group This is a group led and determined by patients, meeting independently of staff with its own agenda and operations. There can be patient councils/forums/groups within inpatient services, day hospitals, residential or community-based services. They are different to users' groups that are separately funded and legal entities in their own right, e.g. charities such as the UK Advocacy Network.

Patient Safety Assessment Process All new NHS CFH products and services are subject to this process, which operates to international standards. The patient safety assessment process is overseen by NHS CFH's national clinical safety officer working with the National Patient Safety Agency. The patient safety assessment process involves three key steps:

1 products are risk-assessed in the context in which they will be used
2 a safety case sets out how identified hazards would be mitigated
3 a safety closure report provides evidence that hazards have been addressed satisfactorily.

Patient's sealed envelope *See* sealing.

Patterns of delivery The way in which services are delivered, their structure and relationship to each other. This does not relate to the content of services.

Payment by Results (PbR)   A funding system for care provided to NHS patients, which pays healthcare providers on the basis of the work they do. It does this by paying a nationally set price or tariff for similar groups of treatments, known as healthcare resource groups (HRG), which itself is based on the historical national average cost of providing services to those HRGs. The fixed tariffs for specified HRGs are set by the DoH and are intended to avoid price differentials across providers that could otherwise distort patient choice. Payment is on a 'per spell' basis, where a spell is defined as a continuous period of time spent as a patient within a trust, and may include more than one episode. The aim of Payment by Results is to provide a transparent, rules-based system for paying NHS trusts. It hopes to reward efficiency, support patient choice and diversity, and encourage strategies for achieving sustainable reductions in waiting times.

Percentage occupancy   Occupied beds expressed as a percentage of the available beds during a given period.

Performance appraisal   A process for assessing performance to assess training needs, job improvement plans and salary reviews, etc.

Performance indicators   A standard of work that acts as a measurement of performance, e.g. response times to requests for work used to indicate the performance of the service. (*See also* quality indicator.)

Performance review   A systematic check on the achievement of the organisation and individuals compared with set objectives.

Perinatal mortality rate   Stillbirths and deaths of infants under one week of age per 1000 total births.

Period of study leave (PSL)   GPs can apply (in accordance with paragraph 50 of the Statement of Fees and Allowances) for financial assistance in connection with a period of study leave to undertake postgraduate education, which will result in benefit to the GP, primary care (in particular) and the NHS.

Permanency planning   Deciding on the long-term future of children who have been moved from their families.

Persistent vegetative state   An irreversible condition resulting from brain damage, characterised by lack of consciousness, thought and feeling, although some reflex activities, such as breathing, continue.

Personal Demographics Service (PDS)   The national electronic database of NHS patient demographic details used within health and social care. Demographic information includes, for example, name, address, date of birth and NHS Number.

Personal Spine Information Service (PSIS) The central database on the Spine containing clinical records for each NHS patient.

Personality The distinctive and identifiable characteristics of an individual human being.

Person specification Derived from the job description and outlines the qualifications, skills and experience required to perform the job. It lists what is essential and what is desirable and it should be used for shortlisting and interviewing. Person specifications should be available and made known to all those considering applying for a post so that they are aware of the criteria that will be used to judge them.

Picture Archiving and Communication Systems (PACS) A system enabling images such as X-rays and scans to be stored and sent electronically so that doctors and other health professionals can access the information with the touch of a button.

Physician's workstation A computer system designed to support the clinical tasks of doctors. (*See also* electronic medical record.)

Planning The process by which the service determines how it will achieve its aims and objectives. This includes identifying the resources which will be needed to meet those aims and objectives.

Police protection The Children Act allows police to detain a child or prevent his or her removal for up to 72 hours if they believe that the child would otherwise suffer significant harm.

Policy An operation statement of intent in a given situation.

Portfolios Personal professional development tools, aimed at encouraging reflection and self-direction in identifying training needs. They record and monitor opportunities for learning and provide tangible evidence of the outcomes. Content varies – for a job interview it will focus on practical skills, competencies and achievements, whereas for academic recognition it will reflect the ability to independently problem solve in the chosen field.

Positive action Measures by which people from particular racial groups are either encouraged to apply for jobs in which they have been under-represented or are given training to help them develop their potential and so improve their chances when competing for particular work.

Postgraduate Education Allowance (PGEA) GPs are eligible if they maintain a balanced programme of education and training geared towards providing the best possible care for their patients. Courses are approved (in advance) by the regional directors of postgraduate general practice education (or their staff) and can be classified in the following three areas: health promotion and prevention; disease management; and service management. GPs have to show that they have attended an average of five days' training a year. Any doctor who does not take part stands to lose financially as they will not be eligible for PGEA. The structure varies and approval may be given for, e.g.:

» lunchtime lecturettes (maybe a half or quarter session)
» in-house practice meetings on specific educational topics
» week-long courses at PG centres (including at overseas resorts)
» national meetings
» reading (free) weekly medical magazines and answering MCQs on the magazine content.

Postscript In computer technology the commercial language that describes a common format for electronic documents that can be understood by printing devices and converted to paper documents or images on a screen.

Practice-based commissioning (PBC) The term given to a form of practice-level commissioning which enables practices (usually this refers to primary care teams led by GPs, although there are some exceptions) to commission care and other services that are directly tailored to the needs of their patients. Practices can keep up to 100% of any savings made by agreement with the local PCT.

Practice parameter *See* clinical guideline.

Preliminary hearing (children) Hearing to clarify matters in dispute, to agree evidence, and to give directions as to the timetable of the case and the disclosure of evidence.

Prescription Pricing Authority (PPA) A national provider of managed services to the NHS. Its main functions are to calculate and make payments for amounts due to pharmacists and GPs for supplying drugs and appliances prescribed under the NHS. It also produces information for NHS organisations and stakeholders about prescribing volumes, trends and costs and manages a range of health benefits, e.g. the NHS Low Income Scheme.

Preventive maintenance and replacement programme A plan for the maintenance of machines to minimise the amount of time lost through breakdown by anticipating and preventing likely problems.

Primary Care Audit Group (i.e. multidisciplinary) Groups of professionals and managers in health authorities whose remit is to encourage and facilitate the undertaking and implementation of audit in primary care – the cyclical reappraisal of structure process and outcome.

Primary care centre (PCC)   Centre for out-of-hours treatment, allowed under changes to the GP contract in 1994.

Primary Care Trust (PCT)   Responsible for commissioning all healthcare in their community.

Principals   Doctors who have been established in general practice by the traditional route, i.e. by means of appointment to the health authorities' GMS Principal List.

Private bed (pay bed)   A bed occupied by a patient who pays the whole cost of accommodation and medical and other services.

Private Finance Initiative (PFI)   Provides a way of funding major capital investments as an alternative to the public procurement route, which is funded directly by the Treasury. Private consortia, usually involving large construction firms, are contracted to design, build, and in some cases manage new projects. Contracts typically last for about 30 years, although some are longer, during which time the building is leased by a public authority. It remains a contentious issue with many critics who state that it does not offer value for money and effectively transfers ownership of NHS hospitals out of the NHS. Others point to the relatively large number of new facilities built under the scheme that would not otherwise have been built.

Private patient   A patient who pays the full cost of all medical and other services.

Probation officer   Welfare professional employed as an officer of the court and financed jointly by the local authority and the Home Office.

Procedure   The steps taken to fulfil a policy. A particular and specified way of doing something.

Professional standards   Professionally agreed levels of performance.

Programmes for IT (PfIT)   Accountability for the delivery of the National Programme for IT (NPfIT) transferred to strategic health authorities on 1 April 2007, as part of the NPfIT Local Ownership Programme (NLOP). The SHAs operate as three Programmes for IT, each of which has a Local Service Provider. These are the London Programme for IT (LPfIT), the Southern Programme for IT (SPfIT) and the North, Midlands and East Programme for IT (NMEfIT).

Prohibited Steps Order (children)   Order that no step which could be taken by a parent in meeting his parental responsibility for a child, and which is of a kind specified in the order, shall be taken by any person without the consent of the court.

Project 2000   The system of nurse education which places increased emphasis on student-centred and research-based learning.

Protocol   The adoption by all staff of local or national guidelines to meet local requirements in a specified way. An alternative word for procedure. (*See also* clinical guideline.)

Provider   A healthcare organisation, such as an NHS trust, which provides healthcare and sells its services to purchasers.

Provider plurality   This term refers to the use of a range of different organisations from NHS and independent, private and 'not-for-profit' sectors in the delivery of services. In the context of NHS reforms, 'provider plurality' coupled with competition and patient choice is said to promote efficiency, effectiveness and value for money in the delivery of services.

PSL   *See* period of study leave.

Psychometric tests   Standardised question and answer papers designed to measure personality.

Public dividend capital (PDC)   A form of long-term government finance on which the NHS trust pays dividends to the government. PDC has no fixed remuneration or repayment obligations, but, in the long term, the overall return on PDC is expected to be no less than on an equivalent loan.

Public Information Programme   *See* Summary Care Record (SCR) Public Information Programme.

Public private partnership (PPP)   The umbrella name given to a range of initiatives which involve the private sector in the operation of public services.

Purchaser   A budget-holding body that buys health or social care services from a provider on behalf of its local population or service users.

Purchasing intelligence   The knowledge purchasers need in order to make informed decisions when purchasing healthcare on behalf of their resident population. Includes demographic data, information on healthcare services, and the views of local people (local voices).

Qualitative reasoning   A subspecialty of artificial intelligence concerned with inference and knowledge representation when knowledge is not precisely defined, e.g. 'back of the envelope' calculations.

Quality   A specified standard of performance.

Quality and Outcomes Framework (QOF)   As part of a new NHS contract, introduced in 2004, GP practices are rewarded for achieving clinical and management quality targets and for improving services for patients within a Quality and Outcomes Framework. It sets out a voluntary system of financial incentives for improving quality within the General Medical Services contract for GP payments.

Quality assurance (QA)   A generic term essentially meaning that one ensures not only that the right things get done, but also that none of the wrong things is done.

Quality improvement strategy   A written statement of objectives relating to quality improvement and a plan for meeting those objectives. The strategy should be consistent with the business plan.

Quality indicator   A standard of service which acts as a measurement of quality, for example incidence of infection used to indicate the quality of care. (*See also* performance indicator.)

Quality Management and Analysis Subsystem (QMAS)   To support the Quality and Outcomes Framework, NPfIT has commissioned British Telecom to develop and implement a new IT system called the Quality Management and Analysis Subsystem. It will provide reporting, forecasting and payment information for improving services within the Quality and Outcomes Framework.

Quango   A quasi-autonomous non-governmental organisation. A body with virtual statutory power.

RA01 Form   Used by a Registration Authority to register a user for access to patient information contained on the Spine. It is made up of two parts:

1   RA01 Part A Form contains the conditions a successful applicant has to agree to prior to becoming an authorised NHS Care Records Service (NHS CRS) user and being issued with a Smartcard

2   RA01 Part B Form is for the registering of users of NHS CRS applications.

Read coding   A hierarchically arranged thesaurus of clinical condition terms which provides a numeric coding system. The system was developed by Dr Read and is cross-referenced to other national and international classifications. Developed initially for primary care medicine in the UK, it was subsequently enlarged and developed to capture medical concepts in a wide variety of situations. (*See also* terminology.)

Reasoning   A method of thinking. (*See also* inference.)

Recovery order (children)   Order which a court can make when there is reason to believe that a child in care, who is the subject of an emergency protection order or in police protection, has been unlawfully taken or kept away from the responsible person, or has run away, is staying away from the responsible person, or is missing.

Recurrent expenditure 'Ongoing expenditure' such as salaries and wages, travelling expenses, drugs and dressings, and provisions.

Reflection The process of returning verbal or body language communication to the original perpetrator to indicate agreement and acceptance.

Refuge (children) Enables 'safe houses' to legally provide care for children who have run away from home or local authority care. A recovery order can be obtained in relation to a child who has run away to a refuge.

Registration Authority Responsible for registering and verifying the identity of individuals who need to access the NHS Care Records Service. After proving their personal identity and being vouched for by a sponsor, the Registration Authority issues staff with a Smartcard and passcode with an approved level of access to patient information.

Regular day admission A patient who attends electively and regularly for a course of treatment and care, but does not stay in hospital through the night.

Relate A voluntary body, formerly known as the Marriage Guidance Council, which assists couples to resolve differences that threaten their relationship.

Representation The method chosen to model a process or object. For example, a building may be represented as a physical scale model, drawing or photograph. (*See also* reasoning and syntax.)

Representations (childcare) *See* complaints procedure.

Research and development (R&D) Searching out knowledge and evidence about the relationship between different factors in the provision of services. Research does not require action in response to findings.

Residential care homes Residential accommodation, other than group homes, providing board and lodging and personal care to the residents. Includes homes for elderly or physically disabled people.

Residential social worker (children) Provides day-to-day care, support and therapy for children living in residential settings, such as children's homes.

Resource assumptions Provisional estimates of cash resources (capital, revenue and joint finance) that may be made available over the next two to three years.

Resource management The different definitions of resource management all emphasise the involvement of doctors, nurses and other clinical staff in the continuing improvement of the quality and quantity of patient care through better use of resources and information.

Respite care   Service giving family members or other carers short breaks from their caring responsibilities.

Responsibility   The obligation that an individual assumes when undertaking delegated functions.

Responsible person (children)   Any person who has parental responsibility for the child, and any other person with whom the child is living. With their consent, the responsible person can be required to comply with certain obligations.

Retainers   Doctors appointed to practices under the Doctors Retainer Scheme who are constrained from practising full-time or part-time usually by virtue of domestic commitments, but who wish to keep in touch with medicine.

Returners   Doctors wishing to return to clinical practice.

Revenue consequences of capital schemes (RCCS)   Annual running costs of capital schemes.

Review   The examination of a particular aspect of a service or care setting so that problem areas requiring corrective action can be identified.

Review (children)   Local authorities have a duty to conduct regular reviews in order to monitor the progress of children they are looking after.

Review meetings   The system whereby the NHSE regional offices monitor the performance of health authorities against planned objectives and set an action plan for further achievements.

Ringfencing   The identification of funds to be used for a particular purpose only – usually applied to funds earmarked by central government for a particular use within the NHS or local government, e.g. the mental illness specific grant.

Risk management   A systematic approach to the management of risk to reduce loss of life, financial loss, loss of staff availability, staff and patient safety, loss of availability of buildings or equipment or loss of reputation.

Risk management strategy   A written statement of objectives for the management of risk and a plan for meeting those objectives. The strategy should be consistent with the business plan.

Role-based access control (RBAC)   Grants a view of a patient's record depending on the role the individual was assigned when they registered for their Smartcard. Authorised users using the NHS Care Records Service will only be able to access the information they need to carry out their role, e.g. a booking clerk will see less information than a doctor.

Safe discharge of patients   A procedure for the discharge of patients who require care in the community which complies with DoH guidelines.

Satisfaction survey   Seeking the views of patients through responses to pre-prepared questions and carried out through interview or self-completion questionnaires.

Sealing   If a patient 'seals' information in their NHS Care Record, it can only be accessed with the patient's agreement, except in exceptional circumstances. Those outside the core team that created the information will see a 'flag' indicating that information is missing.

▶ **Seal and Lock:** If a patient 'seals and locks' information in their NHS Care Record, no one will be able to look at the sealed information outside of the team that added it to the record. Other staff will not be informed that any 'sealed and locked' information exists. Information may be disclosed by the team that recorded it only where the law requires this to save others from serious harm, or where the information has been anonymised so that others will not know who it relates to.

▶ **Clinician Sealed Record:** As now, clinicians can only withhold information from patients permanently in very exceptional circumstances. Those circumstances include where there is a clear danger that the information may cause serious harm to the patient or to someone else, or if it contains confidential information about other people. In those circumstances, it is intended that clinicians will be able to seal information from a patient's view. At the time of writing the process of achieving this is still being considered. Clinicians may also, with the patient's agreement, seal information until they can discuss it with the patient, e.g. an upsetting test result. This is particularly relevant as patients begin to be able to access their own Summary Care Record using HealthSpace. The Data Protection Act exempts clinicians from revealing the information that they have kept from patients for lawful reasons.

▶ **Patient Sealed Record:** Allows a patient to place restrictions on access to parts of their records. (*See also* partial access.)

▶ **Partial access:** As the NHS Care Records Service develops, but not right away, patients will be able to limit access to elements of their record by asking that certain information in the record is hidden from normal view. This will be known as a patient's 'sealed record'. Hidden information will only be accessible with the person's express permission, except in exceptional circumstances. In the future, patients will have two options for sealing information.

Second opinion   An independent opinion from a senior clinician (possibly from another specialty) who has experience of the patient's condition but who is not directly involved in the patient's care. An opinion based on examination of the patient by the clinician.

Secondary Uses Service (SUS)   A single repository of person and care event level data relating to the NHS care of patients, which is used for management and clinical purposes other than direct patient care. These secondary uses include healthcare planning, commissioning, public health, clinical audit, benchmarking, performance improvement, research and clinical governance. The Information Centre for Health and Social Care is working in partnership with NHS Connecting for Health to develop and support the service so that it reflects user needs and requirements and protects patients' rights to confidentiality.

Section 8 orders (children)   The four new orders contained in the Children's Act, which, to varying degrees, regulate the exercise of parental responsibility.

Secure accommodation (children)   Provides for the circumstances in which a child who is being looked after by the local authority can be placed in secure accommodation. Such accommodation is provided for the purpose of restricting the liberty of the child.

Seeding   The process of 'planting' all or part of an idea or plan in the mind(s) of others such that those persons produce the plan as if it were their own original thought.

Semantics   The meaning associated with a set of symbols in a given language, which is determined by the syntactic structure of the symbols, as well as knowledge captured in an interpretative model. (*See also* syntax.)

Seminar   A session during which prepared papers are presented to the class by one or more students.

Sensitively flagged records   Indicates that a demographics record for certain people requires extra protection from unauthorised access, e.g. those in adoption cases and victims of domestic violence. Controls are in place to limit access to patient details that would allow such patients to be contacted. In these cases, the patient's address, telephone numbers and GP registration will not be visible on the Personal Demographics Service.

Service The term used to describe part of an organisation, as opposed to the entire organisation. (*See also* organisation.)

Service contract A legally binding contract between an organisation and an external supplier of goods or services. The contract sets out the agreed cost and quality for a given period.

Service level agreement The term used to describe a document, agreed between organisations or services that will provide and receive a service, which sets out in detail how the service will be provided.

Significant harm (children) 'Whether harm suffered by the child is significant turns on the child's health or development; his [or her] health or development shall be compared with that which could reasonably be expected of a similar child'.

Skill mix The balance of skill, qualifications and experience of nursing and other clinical staff employed in a particular area. The process of reassessing the skill mix required is known as reprofiling.

Slippage The shortfall compared with planned spending caused by delays in the planning or execution of expenditure. Can be expressed in terms of money or time.

Smartcard A plastic card containing an electronic chip (like a chip and PIN credit card) used to identify those who are authorised to use the NHS Care Records Service (NHS CRS). This is used together with an alphanumeric passcode. The chip on the Smartcard does not contain any personal information. It provides a secure link between the NHS CRS and the database holding the user's information and assigned access rights. The Smartcard is printed with the user's name, photo and unique identity number.

Smartcard passcode *See* passcode.

Social worker Generic term applying to a wide range of staff who undertake different kinds of social welfare responsibilities. (*See also* education welfare officer, fieldworker, probation officer and residential social worker.)

Specialty costing The analysis of costs to clinical specialties, thus enabling comparisons to be made in the same institution over time or between different institutions.

Specific Issue Order (children) Order giving directions for the purpose of determining a specific question which has arisen, or which may arise, in connection with any aspect of parental responsibility for a child.

Spine A national, central service that underpins the NHS Care Records Service. It manages the patient's national Summary Care Records. Clinical information is held in the Personal Spine Information Service (PSIS) and demographic information is held in the Personal Demographics Service (PDS). The Spine also supports other systems and services such Choose and Book and the Electronic Prescription Service (EPS).

Spine Directory Services (SDS) The main information source about NHS registered users and accredited systems and services. It ensures that transactions/messages are only processed from authorised users and systems. The Spine Directory Service also stores a record of each NHS organisation. It is a key component of the Spine.

Sponsor A member of staff appointed by an NHS organisation's Executive team to vouch for staff applying for a Smartcard and passcode to gain access to the NHS Care Records Service. Sponsors will usually be a member of staff's operational head, manager or administrator within a practice, clinic, ward or department. They may also be a member of the HR/personnel department.

Staffed allocated beds Staffed beds allocated to particular specialties including those which are available and those which are temporarily not available.

Staff Incident Reporting System A standardised system for reporting incidents and near misses. The NHSE recommends that no more than two types of forms are used for this.

Standardised mortality ratio (SMR) The number of deaths in a given year as a percentage of those expected. The expected number is a standard sex/age mortality of a reference period.

Standing financial instructions Specific instructions issued by the board of a hospital or trust to regulate conduct of the organisation, its directors, managers and agents in relation to all financial matters.

Standing orders A series of established instructions governing the manner in which business will be conducted.

Standards Standards are a means of describing the level of quality that healthcare organisations are expected to meet or to aspire to. The performance of organisations can be assessed against this level of quality.

Strategic Health Authority (SHA) SHAs are responsible for managing the NHS locally and acting as a conduit between NHS organisations and the DoH. They oversee the local implementation of national policy and are responsible for devising overarching local plans for the NHS to improve services and the health of their population. Accountability for the delivery of the National Programme for IT transferred to SHAs in April 2007, as part of the NPfIT Local Ownership Programme (NLOP).

Strategy A long-term plan.

Subject Access Request A written, signed request from an individual to see information held on them by an organisation, made under the Data Protection Act 1998.

Suggestion The process of putting a thought, plan or desire to another person.

Summary Care Record (SCR) A summary of a patient's health information. Patients will, over the next few years, have a Summary Care Record, which will be available to authorised healthcare professionals treating them anywhere in the NHS in England. At first, the information in the Summary Care Record will come from their GP record and will contain their current medications, adverse reactions and allergies. Later, it may be added to from other parts of the NHS. Initially, the Summary Care Record will contain only basic essential information such as current medications and allergies and bad reactions to medicines in the past. Patients will be able to request that sensitive information, for example relating to mental or sexual health, or other matters that they consider sensitive, is restricted.

Summary Care Record (SCR) Public Information Programme A rolling programme to raise public awareness about linking electronic medical records and what it means for patients. The programme began in 2007 in early adopter areas for the Summary Care Record. Information and advice is being provided about how health records will be handled differently and patients' options for participating. It is important to ensure that NHS frontline staff and other patient-facing groups are trained to handle patient queries which may result from the Public Information Programme.

Supervision order (children) Order including, except where express contrary provision is made, an interim supervision order.

Supervisor (children) Person under whose supervision the child is placed by virtue of an order.

Supplier Attachment Scheme (SAS) The Supplier Attachment Scheme is a new opportunity for NHS professionals to have a direct influence on the future of healthcare by working in one of a range of roles with a Local Service Provider.

Supplier Liaison   The function of Supplier Liaison is to assist IT suppliers to locate information on the National Programme and to provide contact details for those organisations that have been awarded contracts.

Supraregional Services   Specialist services for rarer conditions provided for a population significantly larger than that of an English region. They are specially funded.

Survey   The collection of views from a sample of people in order to obtain a representative picture of the views of the total population being studied.

Synchronous communication   A mode of communication when two parties exchange messages across a communication channel at the same time, e.g. telephones. (*See also* asynchronous communication.)

Synergy   The extent to which investment of additional resources produces a return which is proportionally greater than the sum of the resources invested. Sometimes known as the '2+2=5' effect.

Syntax   The rules of grammar that define the formal structure of a language. (*See also* semantics.)

Systematised Nomenclature of Human and Veterinary Medicine (SNOMED)   A commercially available general medical terminology, initially developed for the classification of pathological specimens. (*See also* terminology.)

Targets   Refer to a defined level of performance that is being aimed for, often with a numerical and time dimension. The purpose of a target is to incentivise improvement in the specific area covered by the target over a particular time frame.

Target Allocation   National share of the resources available calculated by reference to established criteria of need.

Team   Any group of people who must significantly relate with each other in order to accomplish shared objectives.

Teleconsultation   Clinical consultation carried out using a telemedical service. (*See also* telemedicine.)

Telemedicine   The delivery of healthcare services between geographically separated individuals, using telecommunication systems, e.g. video conferencing.

Temporarily closed beds   Staffed allocated beds closed for less than one month.

Term In medical terminology an agreed name for a medical condition or treatment. (*See also* code and terminology.)

Terminal A screen and keyboard system that provides access to a shared computer system, e.g. a mainframe or mini-computer. In contrast to computers on a modern network, terminals are not computers in their own right.

Terminology A set of standard terms used to describe clinical activities. (*See also* term.)

T group Training group; refers to training in interpersonal awareness or sensitivity, where a group of people meet in an unstructured way to discuss the interplay of the relationships between them.

Theory X A theory about motivation expounded by Douglas McGregor, which suggests that people are lazy, selfish and unambitious, and need to be treated accordingly. It contrasts with Theory Y, the optimistic view of people.

Theory Z An expression coined by William G. Ouchi as a result of studying Japanese success in industry, to denote a process of organisational adaptation in which the management of the enterprise concentrates on co-ordinating people, not technology, in the pursuit of productivity.

Those close to the patient Anyone nominated by the patient, close relatives (including parents if the patient is a child), partners, close friends, paid or unpaid carers outside the healthcare team and independent advocates. In some circumstances this may include attorneys for property and financial affairs and other legal proxies.

Throughput The number of patients using each bed in a given period, such as a year. (*See also* bed turnover.)

Top slicing Usually used to refer to a proportional sum of money retained from budgets in a district or region to fund, e.g. regionwide initiatives, or supplement financial reserves.

Total Quality Management (TQM) Approach to management of organisations which aims to change organisational culture, so that continuous improvements in quality are achieved, by moving from a traditional command structure to one which encourages and empowers staff.

Training The process of modifying behaviour at work through instruction, example or practice.

Training and Development Strategy A written statement of objectives for the training and development of staff and a plan for meeting these objectives. The strategy should be consistent with the business plan.

Training Needs Analysis An approach to assessing the training or development needs of groups of employees aimed at clarifying the needs of the job and the needs of the individuals in terms of the training required.

Transfer of Undertakings – Protection of Employment (TUPE) A safeguard of employees' rights where businesses change hands between employers.

Transaction Messaging Service A message transfer service that forms part of the Spine. The service allows messages from NHS Care Records Service users to be securely routed to the service they are requesting and to manage the response to that request.

Treatment centre Centres are dedicated units that offer pre-booked day and short-stay surgery and diagnostic procedures in specialties such as ophthalmology, orthopaedics, hernia repair and gallbladder and cataract removal, among others. Treatment centres can be run by the NHS or the Independent Sector and exist mainly to provide additional capacity (including staff) to address waiting list targets.

Tribunal A court-like procedure for the resolution of disputes.

Turing Test Proposed by Alan Turing, the test suggests that an artefact can be considered intelligent if its behaviour cannot be distinguished by humans from other humans in controlled circumstances. (*See also* artificial intelligence.)

Turnover interval The average number of days that beds are vacant between successive occupants.

Tutorial A discussion session, usually dealing with specified content, or a recent lecture or practical. Chaired by the teacher, it may have any number of students from one to 20 or so.

Unbundling and bundling Under the Payment by Results (PbR) system, trusts are reimbursed per spell, categorised by HRG (*see* PbR definition above). There are debates as to whether the HRG categories accurately reflect the cost of providing services, and whether they are flexible enough to incorporate varying treatment patterns. When people refer to 'unbundling' the tariff, they mean being able to clearly identify the individual elements which go to make up the cost of each component of the HRG. This would allow different organisations to carry out different parts of the treatment. For example, unbundling the tariff for an HRG that includes a hospital procedure and after care, means that the after care can be administered in the community, with both the hospital and community provider accurately reimbursed for the work that they do. Conversely, when people talk about 'bundling' the tariff, they mean budgeting for whole patient pathways or treatment programmes, which allows the individual components to be negotiated locally.

Unusual medications Medications which are currently unlicensed or being used for an unlicensed indication. Patients must be informed before they receive such medications.

Underlying deficit This is the total amount of one-off measures the health economy has had to find to achieve a break-even position at year end, i.e. the overall position after ignoring 'in-year' non-recurrent measures.

Valid consent The legal principle by which a patient is informed about the nature, purpose and likely effects of any treatment proposed before being asked to consent to accepting it. (*See also* informed consent.)

Value analysis Also known as value engineering. Term used to describe an analytical approach to the function and costs of every part of a product with a view to reducing costs while retaining the functional ability.

Virement The transfer of resources from one budget heading to another. It is a means of using a planned and agreed saving in one area to finance expenditure in another area. Clear rules are needed about how virement operates so that, for instance, a budget for one-off purchases (e.g. purchase of equipment) is not spent on recurrent payments (e.g. employing staff).

Virtual reality Computer-simulated environment within which humans are able to interact in some manner that approximates interactions in the physical world.

Vital services In management terms those services that are essential to the normal operation of the organisation. Examples include electricity, water, medical gases and telecommunications.

Voice mail Computer-based telephone messaging system, capable of recording and storing messages, for later review or other processing, e.g. forwarding to other users. (*See also* email.)

Waiting list The number of people awaiting admission to hospital as inpatients.

Waiting time The time that elapses between (1) the request by a general practitioner for an appointment and the attendance of the patient at the outpatients' department, or (2) the date a patient's name is put on an inpatients' list and the date they are admitted.

Ward of Court A child who, as the subject of wardship proceedings, is under the protection of the High Court. No important decision can be taken regarding the child while they are a ward of court without the consent of the wardship court.

Wardship   Legal process whereby control is exercised over the child in order to protect the child and safeguard his or her welfare.

Weighted capitation   Sum of money provided for each resident in a particular locality. The three main factors reflected in the formula are: age structure of the population; its morbidity; and relative cost of providing services.

Welfare Checklist (children)   Refers to the innovatory checklist contained in the Children Act.

Welfare Report (children)   The Children Act gives the court the power to request a report on any question in respect of a child under the Act.

Whole-time equivalents (WTEs)   The total of whole-time staff, plus the whole time equivalent of part-time staff, which is obtained by dividing the hours worked in a year by part-timers, by the number of hours in the whole-time working year.

Wide area network (WAN)   Computer network extending beyond a local area such as a campus or office. (*See also* local area network.)

Work in progress   Waiting lists or queues waiting to be seen.

Work Measurement   A work study technique designed to establish the time for a qualified person to carry out a specified job to a defined level.

Work Study   Includes several techniques for examining work in all its contexts, in particular factors affecting economy and efficiency, with a view to making improvements.

Written agreement (children)   Agreement arrived at between the local authority and the parents of children for whom it is providing services. These arrangements are part of the partnership model that is seen as good practice under the Children Act.

Related reading

Some useful sources of further information on these topics are to be found at the following websites.

Department of Health: www.dh.gov.uk

Healthcare Commission: www.healthcare-commission.org.uk

Herzberg F, Mausner B, Snyderman BB. *Herzberg on Motivation*. Cleveland, OH: Penton/IPC; 1983.

Herzberg F, Mausner B, Snyderman BB. *The Motivation to Work*. New York: Wiley; 1959.
King's Fund: www.kingsfund.org.uk
NHS Alliance: www.nhsalliance.org
Royal College of Nursing: www.rcn.org.uk

Useful health-related acronyms

The following list excludes virtually all the clinical acronyms. Fortunately, you don't need to know these acronyms but I felt a reference source might be useful. There has been a burgeoning of acronyms in recent years. I have removed some of the more obvious, such as degrees, diplomas and other medical qualifications and many very common clinical ones. Some have lapsed, although they are still to be found referred to in literature and thus have been included. Interestingly, some have appeared and disappeared in the interval between this and the previous edition! For interest's sake only, included are a handful of mildly amusing ones to be found, although you will need to look carefully for them. I hope that none cause offence, but the author is only reporting those in current use or as reported in current literature.

A
A&C   administrative and clerical
A&E   Accident and Emergency
AA   Attendance Allowance
AAA   Annual Accountability Agreement; abdominal aortic aneurysm
AAC   Advisory Appointments Committee

AAGBI Association of Anaesthetists of Great Britain and Ireland
AAMS Association of Air Medical Services (US)
AAO American Academy of Ophthalmology
AAOS American Academy of Orthopaedic Surgeons
AAOX3 awake, alert and oriented to date, place and person
ABC activity-based costing
ABG arterial blood gases
ABHI Association of British Healthcare Industries
ABI area-based initiative
ABM activity-based management
ABN Association of British Neurologists
ABPI Association of the British Pharmaceutical Industry
ABS Adult Basic Skills
AC Audit Commission
ACA Area Cost Adjustment (part of the SSA)
ACAC Area Clinical Audit Committee
ACAD Ambulatory Care and Diagnostic Centre
ACAS Advisory, Conciliation and Arbitration Service (set up
  by the UK government to assist in the resolution of disputes
  between employers and employees)
ACBS Advisory Committee on Borderline Substances
ACC Adjusted Credit Ceiling (part of capital control framework)
ACCEA Advisory Committee on Clinical Excellence Awards
ACDA Advisory Committee on Distinction Awards (consultants)
ACDC Ambulatory Care and Diagnostic Centre
ACDM Association of Clinical Data Managers
ACDP Advisory Committee on Dangerous Pathogens
ACEVO Association of Chief Executives of Voluntary
  Organisations
ACF Association of Charitable Foundations
ACGT Advisory Committee on Genetic Testing
ACHCEW Association of Community Health Councils for England
  and Wales (now obsolete)
ACHMS Asian Community Mental Health Services
ACIE Association of Charity Independent Examiners
ACIG Academy of Medical Royal Colleges Information Group
ACLS Advanced Coronary Life Support
ACM Assessment and Care Management – Social Services
  community care purchaser division
ACME Advisory Committee on Medical Establishment
  (Scotland); Alliance for Continuing Medical Education

ACMT   Advisory Committee on Medical Training (European); *American College of Medical Toxicology*

ACOST   (Cabinet) Advisory Committee on Science and Technology

ACP   American College of Physicians

ACPC   Area Child Protection Committee

ACR   American College of Radiology

ACRA   (DoH) Advisory Committee on Resource Allocation

ACRA   Advisory Committee on Resource Allocation (obsolete)

ACRPI   Association of Clinical Research for the Pharmaceutical Industry

ACT   Assertive Community Treatment

ACTAF   Association of Community Trusts and Foundations Now Community Foundation Network

ACTR   Additional Cost of Teaching and Research (in Scotland)

ACTS   Agency for Community Team Support

ADA   Americans with Disabilities Act

ADC   automatic data capture

ADCU   Anti-Drugs Co-ordination Unit

ADD   Attention Deficit Disorder

ADH   additional duty hours (junior doctors)

ADHD   Attention Deficit Hyperactivity Disorder

ADI   acceptable daily intake

ADL   activities of daily living

ADMS   Assistant Director of Medical Services

ADNS   Assistant Director of Nursing Services

ADP   automatic data processing

ADQ   average daily quantity (average amount of a medication prescribed for an adult in England)

ADR   adverse drug reaction; alternative dispute resolution

ADS   Attribution Data Set

ADSS   Association of Directors of Social Services

ADSU   Automatic Distress Signal Unit

AED   Automatic External Defibrillator

AEF   Aggregate External Finance

AELS   Advanced Endocrinological Life Support

AEN   Additional Educational Needs (part of SSA)

AES   Assigned Educational Supervisor

AFAIAA   as far as I am aware

A4A   Awards for All

AfC   Agenda for Change

AFOM   Association of the Faculty of Occupational Medicine
AFPP   Association for Perioperative Practice
AFR   annual financial return
AfS   Action for Sustainability
AFWG   Allocation Formula Working Group (part of Home Office)
AGH   Advisory Group on Hepatitis
AGM   annual general meeting
AGMETS   Advisory Group for Medical Education, Training and Staffing (an overarching body designed to co-ordinate all issues relating to staffing and educating doctors)
AGREE   Appraisal of Guidelines for Research and Evaluation in Europe
AGUM   Association for Genito-urinary Medicine
AHA   Associate of the Institute of Hospital Administrators (previously Area Health Authority)
AHCPA   Association of Health Centre and Practice Administrators
AHHRM   Association of Healthcare Human Resource Management
AHP   allied health professional
AHRQ   Agency for Healthcare Research and Quality
AHSC   Academic Health Science Centre
AI   artificial intelligence
AICD   Automatic Internal Cardiac Defibrillator
AIDS   Acquired Immune Deficiency Syndrome
AIF   area investment frameworks
AIM   activity information mapping; advanced informatics in medicine
AIMS   Association for Improvements in Maternity Services
AIOPI   Association of Information Officers in the Pharmaceutical Industry
AIP   approval in principle
ALA   Association of Local Authorities
ALAC   Artificial Limb and Appliance Centre (Now known as the DSC.)
ALARM   Association of Litigation and Risk Managers
ALBs   arm's length bodies
ALD   Adult with Learning Difficulties
ALF   activity-led funding
ALI   Adult Learning Inspectorate
ALM   Action Learning for Managers

ALMO   Arm's Length Management Organisation
ALOS   average length of stay
ALPBs   arm's length public bodies
ALPHA   Access to Learning for the Public Health
ALPHA   Access to Learning for the Public Health Agenda
ALS   Advanced Life Support
ALSOB   alcohol-like substance on breath
AM   Assembly Member (Wales)
AMA   against medical advice; American Medical Association; Association of Metropolitan Authorities
AME   annual managed expenditure
AMEE   Association for Medical Education in Europe
AMIA   American Medical Informatics Association
AMP   annual maintenance plan; asset management plan
AMPS   assessment of motor and process skills
AMQ   average monthly quantities (the assumed maintenance dose per month for an adult of a drug)
AMRA   Asset Management Revenue Account
AMRC   Academy of Medical Royal Colleges; Association of Medical Research Charities
AMS   Army Medical Services
AMSPAR   Association of Medical Secretaries, Practice Administrators and Receptionists
AND   Allow natural death
ANDPB   advisory non-departmental public bodies
ANH   artificial nutrition and hydration
ANP   advanced nurse practitioner
A/O   alert and orientated
AOB   alcohol on breath
AOC   Adult Opportunity Centre
AODP   Association of Operating Department Practitioners (formerly BAODA: British Association of Operating Department Assistants)
AOMRC   Academy of Medical Royal Colleges
AOP   Association of Optometrists
AOT   Assertive Outreach Team
APC   antigen-presenting cell; Area Prescribing Committee
APD   Advanced Professional Development
APH   aged persons home (aka EPH); Association of Public Health (now turned into UKPHA)
APHA   American Public Health Association

APHI Association of Public Health Inspectors
APL accredited prior learning
APLS Advanced Paediatric Life Support
APMS Alternative Primary Medical Services; Alternative Provider Medical Services
A/R alert and responsive
APROP Action for the Proper Regulation of Private Hospitals
APSE Association for Public Service Excellence
AQ Advancing Quality
AQH Association for Quality in Healthcare
AQS Air Quality Strategy
ARC Arthritis and Rheumatism Council
ARCP Annual Review of Competence Progression
ARF Annual Retention Fee
ARG Academic Review Group
ARM Association of Radical Midwives
ARSH Association of Royal Society of Health
ARVAC Association for Research in the Voluntary and Community Sector
AS associate specialist
ASA Ambulance Service Association
ASAP as soon as possible
ASB anti-social behaviour
ASBAH Association for Spina Bifida and Hydrocephalus
ASBO Anti-Social Behaviour Order
ASC Action for Sick Children
ASCT Asylum Seeker Co-ordination Team
ASD Autistic Spectrum Disorder
ASEC Associate Specialist Education Committee
ASGBI Association of Surgeons of Great Britain and Ireland
ASH Action on Smoking and Health
ASIM American Society of Internal Medicine
ASIT Association of Surgeons in Training
ASME Association for the Study of Medical Education
ASPFA Asylum Seekers and People From Abroad (a Social Services team who pay out cash to people who cannot get Social Security Benefits)
ASPIRE Action to Support Practices Implementing Research Evidence
ASSIST Association for Information Management and Technology Staff in the NHS

ASTC Associate Specialist Training Committee
ASTRO-PU Age Sex Temporary Resident Originated Prescribing Unit
ASW Approved Social Worker (A social worker approved to carry out Sections under the Mental Health Act.)
ASWCS Avon Somerset and Wiltshire Cancer Services
ATLS Advanced Trauma Life Support
ATMD Association of Trust Medical Directors
ATU Alcohol Treatment Unit
AUDGP Association of University Departments of General Practice
AURE Alliance of UK Health Regulators on Europe
AVG Ambulatory Visit Group
AvMA Action for Victims of Medical Accidents
AWMEG All-Wales Management Efficiency Group

B

BAAF British Agencies for Adoption and Fostering
BACCH British Association for Community Child Health
BAC blood alcohol content
BACS British Association for Chemical Specialities
BACTS British Association of Clinical Terminology
BACUP British Association of Cancer United Patients
BAEM British Association for Accident and Emergency Medicine
BAMM British Association of Medical Managers (for clinicians in, or interested in, management)
BAMS Benefits Agency Medical Service
BAN British Approved Name
BAO British Association of Otolaryngologists
BAOT British Association of Occupational Therapists
BAP British Association for Psychopharmacology
BAPS British Association of Paediatric Surgeons; British Association of Plastic Surgeons
BAPT British Association of Physical Training
BARQA British Association of Research Quality
BASH British Association for the Study of Headache
BASICS British Association of Immediate Care
BASRaT British Association of Sports Rehabilitators and Trainers
BASSAC British Association of Settlements and Social Action Centres
BASW British Association of Social Workers

BaTA Blood and Transplant Authority
BAUS British Association of Urological Surgeons
BBP blood-borne pathogen
BBS Bulletin Board System
BBV blood-borne virus
BC Block Contract[ing]; Borough Council
BCA Basic Credit Approval (part of capital control framework)
BCCCF Black Community Care Consultative Forum
BCD black and culturally diverse
BCF Boundary Change Factor (part of SSA)
BCHS Better Care Higher Standards
BCODP British Council of Disabled People
BCS British Computer Society
BCSH British Committee for Standards in Haematology
BDA British Dental Association; British Diabetic Association
    (now called Diabetes UK); British Dietetic Association; British
    Dyslexia Association
BDD body dysmorphic disorder
BDH British Drug Houses (no longer trading)
BEAM Biomedical Equipment Assessment and Management
BEHAF British Ethnic Health Awareness Foundation
BGM Board General Manager (an NHS in Scotland term)
BGS British Geriatrics Society for Health in Old Age
BHAF Black HIV and AIDS Forum
BHF British Heart Foundation
BHS British Hypertension Society
BIBRA British Industrial Biological Association
BILD British Institute of Learning Disabilities
BIM British Institute of Management
BioRes Biological and Biomedical Sciences Research (Internet
    resource)
BIR British Institute of Radiology
BIVDA British In Vitro Diagnostics Association
BLROA British Laryngological, Rhinological and Otological
    Association
BLS Basic Life Support
BMA British Medical Association
BMCIS building maintenance cost information system
BME black and minority ethnic
BMI Body Mass Index
BMIS British Medical Informatics Society

BMJ *British Medical Journal*
BMR basal metabolic rate
BNF *British National Formulary* (quarterly publication containing details of prescribed drugs)
BNI British Nursing Index
BOA British Orthopaedic Association
BOPCAS British Official Publications Current Awareness Service
BOS British Orthodontic Society
BP *British Pharmacopoeia*
BPA British Paediatric Association
BPAS British Pregnancy Advisory Service
BPC British Pharmaceutical Codex
BPD borderline personality disorder
BPMF British Postgraduate Medical Federation
BPPV benign paroxysmal positional vertigo
BPR business process re-engineering
BPS British Pharmacological Society
BPSU British Paediatric Surveillance Unit
BR budget requirement
BrAC breath alcohol content
BrAPP British Association of Pharmaceutical Physicians
BRCS British Red Cross Society
BSA Basic Skills Agency
BSAD British Sports Association for the Disabled
BSC Business Service Centre (NHS Wales)
BSCC British Society for Clinical Cytology
BSE bovine spongiform encephalopathy; breast self-examination
BSEC Basic Surgical Education Committee
BSH British Society for Haematology
BSI British Society for Immunology; British Standards Institution
BSL British Sign Language
BSPED British Society for Paediatric Endocrinology and Diabetes
BSR British Society of Rheumatology
BSS basic surgical skills
BST basic surgical training; basic specialist training
BSTC Basic Surgical Training Committee; Basic Surgical Training Course
BSVP Better Services for Vulnerable People
BTEG Black Training and Enterprise Group

BTS   Blood Transfusion Service; British Thoracic Society
BUPA   British United Provident Association
BVACoP   Best Value Accounting Code of Practice
BVPI   Best Value Performance Indicator
BVPP   Best Value Performance Plan
BWS   Beached Whale Syndrome

C

CAB   Citizens Advice Bureau
CABA   Compressed Air Breathing Apparatus
CABE   Commission for Architecture and the Built Environment
CABG   Coronary Artery Bypass Graft
CADO   Chief administrative dental officer
CAEF   Clinical Audit and Effectiveness Forum
CAF   Charities Aid Foundation
CAFCASS   Children And Family Court Advisory Support
Service
CAIT   Citizens Advocacy Information and Training
CAL   Computer assisted learning
CALL   Cancer Aid Listening Line
CAM   Complementary and Alternative Medicine
CAMHS   Child & Adolescent Mental Health Services – Joint
Local and Health Authority services to young people with
mental health problems.
CAMO   Chief administrative medical officer
CAMS   Computer Aided Medical Systems
CAN   Community Action Network
CANH   Clinically assisted nutrition and hydration
CANO   Chief Area Nursing Officer
CAOX4   conscious, alert/awake and orientated to person, place,
time and recent events
CAP   College of American Pathologists
CAPD   Continuous Ambulatory Peritoneal Dialysis for people with
kidney failure
CAPM   Capital Asset Pricing Model
CAPO   Chief administrative pharmaceutical officer
CARE   Clinical Audit and Research Evidence; Craniofacial
Anomalies Register
CAS   Controls assurance statement; Care Assessment Schedule;
Chemical Abstracts; Community Accountancy Service;
Controls Assurance Statement

CASE Centre for Analysis of Social Exclusion

CASH Consensus Action on Salt and Health

CASP Critical Appraisal Skills Programme

CASPE Clinical Accountability Service Planning and Evaluation Specialist Healthcare Training Group

CAT Computerised axial tomography; Critically Appraised Topic; Community Alcohol Team

CATS Credit Accumulated Transfer Scheme (a national scheme)

CAWG Controls Assurance Working Group

CBA cost-benefit analysis; competence-based assessment

CbD case-based discussion

CBRN Chemical, Biological, Radioactive and Nuclear

CBS Common basic specification

CBT Cognitive Behavioural Therapy; Computer Based Training

CC Charity Commission; County Council; Chief Complaint; City Council

CCA Cost-Consequence Analysis; Current Cost Accounting

CCC NHS Centre for Coding and Classification.

CCCG Cochrane Colorectal Cancer Group

CCDC Consultant in Communicable Disease Control

CCE Completed consultant episode (*see* FCE)

CCEPP Cochrane Collaboration on Effective Professional Practice – now called EPOC

CCETSW Central Council for Education and Training in Social Work (abolished October 2001)

CCG Community Care Grant

CCHR Citizens Commission on Human Rights

CCIT Consultant Contract Implementation Team

CCN County Councils' Network; Change Control Notice

CCP Community Care Plan; Change Control Procedure

CCR Cross Cutting Review

CCrISP Care of the Critically Ill Surgical Patient

CCRN Comprehensive Clinical Research Network

CCSC Central Consultants and Specialists Committee (a committee of BMA)

CCSI Critical Care Skills Institute

CCSR Cross Cutting Spending Review

CCST Certificate of completion of specialist training for junior doctors

CCT Certificate of Completion of Training; compulsory

competitive tendering (a sort of Dutch auction of public services, now partly replaced by the Best Value process)

CCTR Cochrane Controlled Trials Register

CCTV Closed Circuit TeleVision

CCU coronary care unit; critical care unit

CD Clinical Director; Clinical Directorate; Controlled Drug; Civil Defence; Cluster of Differentiation

CDC Center for Disease Control and Prevention (USA)

CDDS Council of Deans of Dental Schools

CDER Center for Drug Evaluation and Research (USA)

CDHN Community Development and Health Network

CDM Chronic disease management; Construction, Design and Management

CDO Chief dental officer

CDS Contract Data Set – A collection of information recorded by the NHS Trust that identifies a patient and their treatment which is sent to the Health Authority; Community Dental Service

CDSC Communicable Disease Surveillance Centre

CDSM Committee on Dental and Surgical Materials (abolished 1994)

CDSR Cochrane Database of Systematic Reviews

CDU Child Development Unit; Central Delivery Unit; Colourflow Duplex Ultrasound

CDX Community Development Exchange

CE chief executive

CEA cost-effectiveness analysis

CEAC Clinical and Excellence Awards Committee (Northern Ireland)

CEDP Chief Executive Development Programme

CEEU Clinical Effectiveness and Evaluation Unit of the RCP

CEF Community Empowerment Fund

CEFET Central England Forum for European Training

CEMACH Confidential Enquiry into Maternal and Child Health, evolved into the Centre for Maternal and Child Enquiries (CMACE).

CEMD Confidential Enquiry into Maternal Deaths

CEMVO Council of Ethnic Minority Voluntary Sector Organisations

CEN Comite Europeen de Normalisation (European Standards organisation)

CEN   Community Empowerment Network
CEO   chief executive officer
CEPOD   Confidential Enquiry into Peri-operative Deaths (*see* NCEPOD)
CERA   Capital Expenditure, Revenue Account
CERES   Consumers for Ethics in Research
CertHSM   Certificate in Health Services Management
CES   Charities Evaluation Services
CESDI   Confidential Enquiry into Stillbirths and Deaths in Infancy
CESH   National Confidential Inquiry into Suicide and Homicide By People With Mental Illness
CEX   Clinical Evaluation Exercise
CF   Cystic Fibrosis
CfH   Connecting for Health
CfI   Centre for Infections (part of HPA)
CFI   Community Finance Initiative
CFISSA   Centrally Funded Initiatives and Services and Special Allocations
CFN   Community Foundation Network
CFO   Chief Finance Officer; Conventionally Financed Option; Co-Financing Public Sector Intermediary Organisation
CfPS   Centre for Public Scrutiny
CFR   Capital Financing Reserve
CFRC   Children and Family Resource Centre
CFS   Chronic Fatigue Syndrome closely associated with ME
CFSMS   Counter Fraud and Security Management Service
CG   Clinical Governance
CGD   Chronic Granulomatous Disease
CGF   Child Growth Foundation
CGRDU   Clinical Governance Research and Development Unit
CGST   Clinical Governance Support Team
CHAI   Commission for Healthcare Audit and Improvement (obs now HC)
CHAIN   Contact Help Advice and Information Network
CHAOS   Chief Has Arrived on the Scene
CHART   Community Health Action Resource Team
CHC   Community Health Council (now only in Wales)
CHCP   community health and care partnership (Scotland)
CHD   coronary heart disease
CHDGP   Collection of Health Data from General Practice project
CHEST   Combined Higher Education Software Team

CHEX   Community Health Exchange
CHFG   Clinical Human Factors Group
CHG   Community Hospitals Group (now taken over by BUPA)
CHI   Commission for Health Improvement; community health index
CHIA   Comprehensive Health Impact Assessment
CHIME   Centre for Health Informatics in Medical Education
CHiQ   Centre for Health Information Quality (patient information)
CHIR   Canadian Institutes of Health Research
CHIRP   Confidential Human Factors Incident Reporting Procedure
CHMS   Council for Heads of Medical Schools; central health and miscellaneous services
CHMU   Central Health Monitoring Unit (obsolete)
CHOU   Central Health Outcomes Unit
CHP   Community Health Partnership (Scotland); Combined Heat and Power
CHRC   Community Health and Resource Centres
CHRE   Council for Healthcare Regulatory Excellence
CHRE   The Council of Healthcare Regulatory Excellence
CHS   child health surveillance
CHS   Community Health Services; Child Health Surveillance
CHSA   Chest, Heart and Stroke Association
CI   Clinical Indicator
CIA   Chief Internal Auditor
CIC   Common Information Core; Charitable Incorporated Organisation
CIM   Capital Investment Manual
CIMP   Clinical Information Management Programme
CIMS   Coalition for Improving Maternity Services
CINAHL   Cumulative Index to Nursing and Allied Health
CIO   Confederation of Indian Organisations; Charitable Incorporated Organisation; Chief Information Officer
CIP   Cost Improvement Programme
CIP(S)   Capital Investment Programme(s)
CIPC   Centre for Innovation in Primary Care
CIPFA   Chartered institute of Public Finance and Accountancy
CIS   Clinical Information System
CISH   Confidential Inquiry into Suicide and Homicide by people with mental illness

CISP Community Information Systems Project

CJC Commissioning Joint Committee

CJD Creutzfeld Jacob Disease

CKD Chronic Kidney Disease

CLA Commissioner for Local Administration (the ombudsman)

CLAPA Cleft Lip and Palate Association

CLDT Community Learning Disability Team

CLGMS Cash Limited General Medical Services

CLib Cochrane Library

CLIP Central-Local Information Partnership; Clinical Improvements Database

CM community midwife

CMA Cost Minimisation Analysis

CMACE Centre for Maternal and Child Enquiries

CMAJ Canadian Medical Association Journal

CMB Central Midwives Board

CMC Central Manpower Committee (no longer exists)

CMD Continuing Medical Development

CMDS contract/core minimum data set

CME continuing medical education

CMF Capital Modernisation Fund

CMHN community mental handicap nurse (obsolete)

CMHSD Centre for Mental Health Services Development, Kings College London

CMHT Community mental health team

CML Chronic Myeloid Leukaemia

CMMS Case mix management system

CMO Chief Medical Officer; (DoH) Corporate Management Board

CMP Civilian Medical Practitioner

CMPS Centre for Management and Policy Studies

CMR Computerised Medical Record

CMS Community Midwifery Service; clinical management support; contract management system

CMT Corporate Management Team

CN charge nurse

CNM clinical nurse manager

CNO chief nursing officer

CNS clinical nurse specialist; community nursing service; central nervous system

CNST Clinical Negligence Scheme for Trusts

CO Cabinet Office; Course Organiser; Complains Of; Chief Officer; Capital Out-turn

COAD Chronic Obstructive Airways Disease – usually called COPD

COGIT Chief Officers' Group of Information Technology

COGPED Committee of General Practice Education Directors

COI Central Office of Information

COIN Circulars on the Internet (e.g. all the Health Service Publications available online as letters, regulations, circulars, CMO updates, advance letters etc.; Clinical Oncology Information Network)

COMA Committee on Medical Aspects of Food Policy (abolished 2000)

COMARE Committee on Medical Aspects of Radiation in the Environment

COMEAP Committee On the Medical Effects of Air Pollutants

COPC Community Oriented Primary Care

COPD Chronic Obstructive Pulmonary Disease

COPDEND Conference of Postgraduate Dental Deans and Directors of Education

COPE Committee on Publication Ethics

COPMED Conference of Postgraduate Medical Deans

COR Capital Out-turn & Receipts return

CORE Clinical Outcomes Research and Effectiveness

COREC Central Office for Research Ethics Committees

COSHH Control of Substances Hazardous to Health Legislation (1994 Regulations)

COSLA Convention of Scottish Local Authorities

COT Committee on Toxicity

CP Community Plan; Cerebral palsy

CPA Care Programme Approach (patients needs for care are assessed on a four point scale: Level 4 means that you are dangerously ill and need supervision; Level 1 means that you are not thought to need anything more than a bit of advice and counselling); Comprehensive Performance Assessment; Clinical Pathology Accreditation; critical path analysis

CPAG Child Poverty Action Group; Capital Prioritisation Advisory Group

CPAP Continuous Positive Airway Pressure

CPC Cost Per Case

CPCCH Consultant Paediatrician in Community Child Health

CPCME   Centre for Postgraduate and Continuing Medical Education

CPCU   Child Protection Co-ordination Unit

CPD   continuing professional development

CPEP   Clinical Practice Evaluation Programme

CPFA   Charted Public Finance Accountant

CPH   Certificate in Public Health

CPHL   Central Public Health Laboratory

CPHM   Certified Professional in Healthcare Materiel Management

CPHMCH   Committee Public Health Medicine and Community Health

CPHVA   Community Practitioners and Health Visitors Association – part of AMICUS

CPMP   Committee for Proprietary Medical Products (EU)

CPN   community psychiatric nurse

CPNA   Community Psychiatric Nurses Association – now the Mental Health Nursing Association

CPO   chief pharmaceutical officer

CPOD   Centre for Professional and Organisational Development

CPPIH   Commission for Patient and Public Involvement in Health (obsolete)

CPR   Child Protection Register; cardiopulmonary resuscitation; Capital Payments & Receipts return

CPS   Child Protection Services

CPSM   Council for Professions Supplementary to Medicine

CPU   Contracts & Purchasing Unit; central processing unit

CPWP   Capital Programmes Working Party

CQC   Care Quality Commission

CQI   Continuous quality improvement

CQSW   Certificate of Qualification of Social Work (abolished 1989)

CQUIN   Commissioning for Quality and Innovation

CQUIN AQ   Commissioning for Quality and Innovation Advancing Quality

CRAG   Clinical Research and Audit Group; Charging for Residential Accommodation Guide – guidance for local authorities on community care financial assessment; Clinical Resource and Audit Group – the lead body within the Scottish Executive Health Department promoting clinical effectiveness in Scotland

CRAGPE   Committee of Regional Advisers in General Practice Education

CRAGPIE   Committee of Regional Advisers in General Practice Education

CRANE   Craniofacial Anomalies Register

CRB   Criminal Records Bureau

CRC   Clinical Research Centre; Cancer Research Campaign

CRCF   Conference of Royal Colleges and their Faculties

CRD   Centre for Reviews and Dissemination

CRDB   Care Record Development Board

CRDC   Central Research and Development Committee

CRE   Commission for Racial Equality (monitors the effects of the Race Relations Act 1976)

CRED   Clinical Governance/Education and R&D subgroup

CRES   Cash Releasing Efficiency Savings

CRHP   Council for the Regulation of Healthcare Professionals (replaced by Council for Healthcare Regulatory Excellence [CHRE])

CRIO   Chief Registration & Inspection Officer – responsible for the Health and Social Service Registration and Inspection Units and Guidance-ad-Litem service

CRIR   Committee for Regulating Information Requirements

CRMD   Cochrane Review Methodology Database

CRT   Community Rehabilitation Team; Cathode Ray Tube

CS   Capital Strategy

CSA   Child Support Agency; Common Services Agency; Clinical Spine Application

CSAG   Clinical Standards Advisory Group

CSASHS   Common Services Agency for the Scottish Health Service

CSBS   Clinical Standards Board for Scotland

CSC   Community Sector Coalition; Computer Sciences Corporation

CSCI   Commission for Social Care Inspection

CSD   carbonated soda drinks

CSEC   Corporate Specialist Education Committee

CSF   Community Support Framework; Cerebro-spinal Fluid

CSM   Committee on Safety of Medicines; Christian Socialist Movement

CSMC   Civil Service Management Committee

CSO   Central Statistical Office; Civil Society Organisation (or NGO)

CSP Chartered Society of Physiotherapy; Children's Services Plan
CSPG Central Support Protection Grant
CSR Comprehensive Spending Review
CSS Children's Social Services; Certificate of Satisfactory Service; Cascading Style Sheets
CSSD Central Sterile Services/Supplies Department; Central Support Service Department
CSTC Corporate Specialist Training Committee
CSV Community Service Volunteers
CT computerised tomography
CTBSL Council Tax Benefit Subsidy Limitation
CTD close to death; circling the drain
CTG cardiotocography electronic measurement of foetal heart and uterine contractions
CTN Charity Trustees Network
CTO Compulsory Treatment Order
CTPLD Community Team for People with Learning Disabilities
CU Casualties Union
CUA Cost-Utility Analysis
CUE Community Unit for the Elderly
CUV current use value
CVCP Committee of Vice Chancellors and Principals
CVE Continuous Vocational Education
CVS Council for Voluntary Service; Cardiovascular system
CYA cover your arse
CYPF Children and Young People's Fund
CYPS Children and Young People's Services
CYPU Children and Young People's Unit

D

D&T drugs and therapeutics
D&TP *Drugs and Therapeutic Bulletin*
DA distributable amount; district audit
DAAT Drug and Alcohol Team
DAN Disabled People's Direct Action Network
DANS duty assessment nurses
DAP Deans Advisory Panel
DARE Database of Abstracts of Reviews of Effectiveness
DART Drug and Alcohol Resistance Training
DASG Drugs and Alcohol Specific Grant
DASS Director of Adult Social Services

DAT   digital audio tape; Disability Appeal Tribunal (obsolete); Drugs Action Team

DATA   Distress Awareness Training Agency

DB   database

D/C   discharge; discontinue

DCLG   Department for Communities and Local Government

DCT   Disabled Children's Team

DCFS   Directorate of Counter Fraud Services

DDA   Disability Discrimination Act 1995; Disabled Drivers' Association

DDD   defined daily dose

DDPHRCS   Diploma in Dental Public Health, Royal College of Surgeons of England

DDRB   Doctors' and Dentists' Review Body (also known as the Review Body on Doctors' and Dentists' Remuneration)

DEB   Dental Estimates Board

DEC   Development and Evaluation Committee (replaced by NICE in 2000)

DEFRA   Department for Environment, Food and Rural Affairs

DEL   Departmental Expenditure Limit

DENS   Doctor's Educational Needs

DFBO   design, finance, build and operate

DfEE   Department for Education and Employment (now renamed DfES)

DfES   Department for Education and Skills

DFT   Distance from Target (relating to HA's financial allocation)

DFFP   Diploma of Faculty of Family Planning

DFG   Disabled Facilities Grant

DG5   The Public Health part of the European Union

DGH   district general hospital

DGM   district general manager

DH   Department of Health (England) (*see* DoH)

DHA   district health authority (obsolete April 2002)

DHSC   Directorate of Health and Social Care (obsolete)

DHSS   Department of Health and Social Security (later split into DoH and DSS)

DHSSPS   Department of Health, Social Services and Public Safety

DHT   District Handicap Team

DI   Director of Information

DIA   Drug Information Association

DIAL   Disablement Information and Advice Lines

DIC   dead in car; disseminated intravascular coagulation
DID   dissociative identity disorder
DIG   Disablement Income Group
DIO   district immunisation officer
DIPEx   Database of Individual Patient Experiences
DIPG   Drug Information Pharmacists Group
DIPHSM   Diploma in Health Services Management
DipSW   Diploma in Social Work
DIS   Departmental Investment Strategy
DisCASS   Disabled Citizens Advice and Support Service
DISP   Developing Information System for Purchasers
DISS   Disability Information Service Surrey
DLA   Disability Living Allowance
DLCV   drugs of limited clinical value
DLF   Disabled Living Foundation
dm+d   Dictionary of Medicines and Devices
DMARD   disease modifying anti-rheumatic drug
DMC   district medical committee
DMD   Drug Misuse Database; Duchenne muscular dystrophy
DMF   Disabled Motorists Federation
DMFT   (number of) decayed, missing, filled teeth
DMHE   Department of Mental Health for the Elderly
DMO   district medical officer (obsolete)
DMT   Departmental Management Team
DMU   directly managed unit
DN   district nurse
DNA   did not arrive; did not attend
DNA-CR   Do not attempt cardiopulmonary resuscitation
DNAR   Do not attempt resuscitation
DNDRN   Dementias and Neurodegenerative Disease Research Network
DNGNet   Disability Network Group
DNI   do not intubate (similar to DNR)
DNR   do not resuscitate
DNS   director of nursing services
DNW   Drugs North West
DOA   date of accident (in A&E departments); date of admission; dead on arrival
DOB   date of birth
DoF   Director of Finance
DOGPE   Director of General Practice Education

DoH   Department of Health
DOPS   Direct Observation of Procedural Skills
DPB   Dental Practice Board (obsolete)
DPC   Data Protection Commissioner
DPGPE   Director of Postgraduate GP Education
DPH   Director of Public Health
DPI   Disabled Peoples' International
DPR   Data Protection Registrar; directorate performance
  review
DPTC   Disabled Person's Tax Credit (now abolished)
DRC   depreciated replacement cost; Disability Rights
  Commission
DRF   direct revenue funding
DRG   diagnosis/diagnostic related group
DRS   Dental Reference Service
DSC   Directory of Social Change; Disablement Service Centre
DSCA   Defence Secondary Care Agency
DSCN   Data Set Change Notice
DSD   Decontamination Services Department
Dsh   deliberate self harm
DSL   Doctors' Support Line
DSO   Direct Service Organisation
DSON   Detailed Statement of Need
DSPD   dangerous and severe personality disorder
DSS   decision support systems; Department of Social Security
  (now the DWP)
DSU   day surgery unit
DTA   Development Trusts Association
DTB   Drug and Therapeutic Bulletin
DTC   Day Treatment Centre; Diagnostic and Treatment Centre;
  Drug and Therapeutics Committee
DTD   document type definition
DTF   Diversity Task Force
DTI   Department of Trade and Industry
DTNI   daytime net inflow
DTTO   Drug Testing and Treatment Order
DTP   Diphtheria Tetanus Pertussis (a vaccine)
DUI   driving under the influence
DV   deo volente (God willing); dependent variable; domestic
  violence; domiciliary visit (by consultant)
DVTA   Dental Vocational Training Authority (obsolete)

DWA Disability Working Allowance (a benefit for people working at least 16 hours a week who have a disability affecting their working ability, now replaced by DPTC)

DWM dead white male

DWP Department for Work and Pensions

E

EAC estimated annual cost

EAG Expert Advisory Group

EAGA Expert Advisory Group on AIDS

EAN European article number

EAPN European Anti Poverty Network

EASR European age standardised rate (a measure of the incidence of disease)

EBD emotional and behavioural difficulties

EBH evidence-based healthcare

EBL evidence-based learning

EBM evidence-based medicine

EBMH evidence-based mental health

eBNF The BNF on CD-ROM

EBOC evidence based on call

EBP evidence-based practice

EBS Emergency Bed Service (London)

EBV Epstein-Barr virus

EC European Community; Experience Corps

ECCA English Community Care Association

ECDL European Computer Driving Licence

ECN Emergency Care Network

ECP Emergency Care Practitioner

ECR Extra-contractual Referral (now replaced by OATS)

ECTS European credit transfer scheme

ED economic development; enumeration district (the smallest unit for census data – about 200 homes)

EDA Erectile Dysfunction Association

EDI electronic data interchange (exchanging information electronically, not including faxing)

EDIFACT Electronic Data Interchange for Administration, Commerce and Transport (Electronic Data Interchange is a particular structure which complies with ISO 9735; this is the standard for EDI adopted by the NHS)

EDIT Elderly Dementia Intervention Team

EDP Education Development Plan; emotionally disturbed person
EDS Ehlers-Danlos syndrome
EDT Emergency Duty Team (Social Services Departments)
EEA European Economic Area
EEC European Economic Community
EFGCP European Forum for Good Clinical Practice
EFL external financing limit
EFM electronic foetal monitoring
EFMI European Federation for Medical Informatics
EFQM European Foundation for Quality Management
EGFR epidermal growth factor receptor; estimated glomerular filtration rate
eGIF Electronic Government Interoperability Framework
EHMA European Healthcare Management Association
EHO environmental health officer
EHP Education and Health Partnership
EHR electronic health record
EHS extremely hazardous substance
EIA European Information Association
EL Executive Letter (has year and number with it)
eLIB Electronic Libraries Programme
ELP Essential Lifestyles Planning (person-centred planning tool emphasising rhythms and routines of daily life used in Learning Disability Services)
EM electronic mail (email)
EMA Education Maintenance Allowance; emergency medical admission
EMAG Ethnic Minority Achievement Grant
EMAS Employment Medical Advisory Service
EMEA European Medicines Evaluation Agency
EMG electromyogram
EMI elderly mentally ill; elderly mentally infirm
EMIS Egton Medical Information System
EMLC European Midwives Liaison Committee
EMO Examining Medical Officer
EMR electronic medical record
EMS emergency medical services
EMW early morning wakening
EMWA European Medical Writers Association
ENB English National Board for Nursing, Midwifery and Health Visiting (obsolete)

ENDPB executive non-departmental public bodies
ENHPA European Network of Health Promotion Agencies
ENIL European Network on Independent Living
ENP emergency nurse practitioner
EO Employers' Organisation
EOC Equal Opportunities Commission (set up under the Sex
 Discrimination Act 1975 to monitor sex discrimination)
EP emergency planning; English Partnerships
EPACT Electronic Prescribing Analysis and Costs
EPCS Environmental, Protective and Cultural Services
EPH elderly persons' home
EPHR electronic patient health record
EPICS Elderly Persons Integrated Care Scheme
EPO emergency planning officer
EPP Expert Patient Programme
EPR electronic patient record
EQUIP Education and Quality in Primary Care; Effectiveness and
 Quality in Practice Group (within DoH, chaired by CMO and
 CNO)
ERA-ETDA European Renal Association-European Dialysis and
 Transplant Association
ERDIP Electronic Record Development Implementation
 Programme
ERG electroretinogram
ERI Edinburgh Research and Innovation Limited
ERIC Estates Returns Information Collection
EROS Electronic Records in Office Systems
ERS External Reference Group (relating to NSFs)
ES educational supervisor; Employment Service
ESAT Emergency Services Action Team (obsolete)
ESF Education Standards Fund; European Social Fund
ESMI elderly severely mentally infirm or ill
ESOL English for speakers of other languages
ESP Economic and Social Partnership
ESRA European Society of Regulatory Affairs (now TOPRA)
ESRC Economic and Social Science Research Council
ESRI Economic and Social Research Institute (Ireland)
ESV Employer Supported Volunteering
ET environmental technologies; executive team
ETA estimated time of arrival
ETF Environment Task Force

ETP   electronic transmission of prescription; Employer Training Pilot
ETT   endotracheal tube
EU   European Union
EWC   expected week of confinement
EWO   educational welfare officer
EWTD   European Working Time Directive
EYDCP   Early Years Development and Childcare Plan
EYDP   Early Years Development Partnership
EYPD   Early Years and Play Department
EYST   Early Years Surgical Training
EZ   Employment Zone

F

FA   Friedreich's ataxia
FAB   Family Action Benchill
FACS   Fair Access to Care Services
FAM   Fraud Awareness Month (an annual event)
FAQs   frequently asked questions
FARR   Fixed Asset Restatement Reserve
FAWN   Funding Advice Workers Network
FBC   full business case
FC   factor cost; family credit (now replaced by tax credits); fixed cost
FCAS   Federation of Charity Advice Services
FCDL   Federation for Community Development Learning
FCE   finished consultant episode (*see* CCE)
FCS   financial control system
FDA   US Food and Drug Administration
FDIU   foetal death in utero
FDL   finance directorate letter
FDTL   Fund for the Development of Teaching and Learning
FE   further education
FEC   Further Education College
FEFC   Further Education Funding Council (disbanded 2001, replaced by the Learning and Skills Council)
FENTO   Further Education National Training Organisation
FES   Family Expenditure Survey
FESC   Framework for Procuring External Support for Commissioning
FFCE   first finished consultant episode

FFP   fresh frozen plasma
FHom   Faculty of Homeopathy
FHR   foetal heart rate
FHS   Family Health Services (the primary healthcare providers, including GPs, dentists, pharmacists and opticians)
FHSA   Family Health Service Authority (role now taken over by the Health Authority)
FHSAA   Family Health Services Appeal Authority
FHSCU   Family Health Services Computer Unit
FHT   foetal heart tones
FIAC   Federation of Independent Advice Centres
FIBD   found in bed dead
FIG   Food Initiatives Group
FIP   financial information project
FIPO   Federation of Independent Practitioner Organisations
FIS   Family Income Supplement (became WFTC); Financial Information Service (run by IPF); financial information system
FIT   Focused Individualised Training
FITTA   fixed-term training appointment
FIU   Fraud Investigation Unit
FM   facilities management
FMD   foot and mouth disease
FMIP   financial management information project
FMIS   financial management information systems
FMP   financial management programme
FMR   functions and manpower review
FOM   Faculty of Occupational Medicine of Royal College of Physicians
FORD   found on road dead
FP10   a prescription form
FPA   Family Planning Association
FPC   Family Planning Clinic; Family Practitioner Committee (which was replaced by the FHSA)
FPharmM   Faculty of Pharmaceutical Medicine
FPHM   Faculty of Public Health Medicine
FPS   Family Planning Services; Family Practitioner Services
FR   financial regulation
FRED   Financial Reporting Exposure Draft (draft FRS)
FRS   Fellow of the Royal Society; Financial Reporting Standard
FRSH   Fellow of the Royal Society of Health
FSA   Financial Services Authority; Food Standards Agency

FSID Foundation for the Study of Infant Deaths
FSM free school meals
FSO Forum Support Organisations
FSS Forensic Science Service
FSSA Federation of Surgical Speciality Associations
FSU Family Support Unit (now known as Family Unit – FU).
FT NHS foundation trust; full-time
FTC Federal Trade Commission
FTE full-time equivalent
FTP fitness to practice
FTR Foundation Training Report
FTSTA Fixed Term Specialty Training Appointment
FTTA Fixed Term Training Appointments
FU Family Unit (a mixture of residential and outreach service for children and young people and their families); follow-up
FWATAG Flexible Working and Training Advisory Group
FWN further work needed
FY full year
FY1 Foundation Year 1
FY2 Foundation Year 2
FYC full-year cost
FYE full-year effect; full-year equivalent

G

GAAP Generally Accepted Accounting Practice
GAD Government Actuary's Department
GAG getting ahead of the game
GAL guardian *ad litem* (usually an independent social worker)
GALRO Guardian Ad Litem Reporting Officer (these are appointed to represent the best interests of the child)
GAPS Genetic Information and Patient Services
GATB Global Alliance for TB Drug Development
GATS General Agreement on Trade in Services
GBP pounds sterling (for people who don't have a £ sign on their computer, etc.)
GBS Guillain-Barré syndrome
G-CAT Government IT Catalogue
GCC General Chiropractic Council
GCS Glasgow Coma Score
GCSE General Certificate of Secondary Education
GDA guideline daily amount

GDC General Dental Council
GDP general dental practitioner; gross domestic product
GDS general dental services
GENECIS General Clinical Information System
GHG General Healthcare Group
GHQ General Health Questionnaire
GHS General Household Survey
GIDA Government Intervention in Deprived Areas
GIGO garbage in, garbage out
GIS Geographical Information System (computers designed to create, manipulate, analyse and display geographical data)
GLACHC Greater London Association of Community Health Councils
GLAD Greater London Association of Disabled People
GLADD Gay and Lesbian Association of Doctors and Dentists
GM Geiger-Muller; general manager
GMC General Medical Council
GMCDP Greater Manchester Coalition of Disabled People
GMO genetically modified organisms
GMP general medical practitioner; good medical practice
GMS general medical services
GMSC General Medical Services Committee
GNP gross national product
GNVQ General National Vocational Qualifications
GO Government Office for the Regions
GOC General Optical Council; Gynaecological Oncology Centre
GOK God only knows
GOMER get out of my emergency room (US slang for an unwelcome patient)
GOP General Optical Council
GOS General Ophthalmic Service
GOSC General Osteopathic Council
GOSH Great Ormond Street Hospital for Children
GP general practitioner; Green Paper
GP2GP the transfer of electronic patient records from one GP to another when a patient changes practices
GPAS General Practice Assessment Survey (produced by the NPCRDC)
GPASS General Practice Administration System Scotland
GPC General Practitioners Committee
GPCC GP Commissioning Consultant

GPCG   GP Commissioning Group (*see* HSC 1998/030)
GPEC   GP Emergency Centre
GPFC   General Practice Finance Corporation
GPFH   General Practitioner Fundholder (obsolete)
GPIAG   General Practice Airways Group
GPMSS   General Practice Minimum System Specification
GPPS   General Professional Practice of Surgery (manual that replaces MBST)
GPR   General Practice Registrar
GPWA   GP Writers Association
GPWSI   GPs with a special interest
GRE   grant related expenditure (replaced by NRE)
GREA   Grant Related Expenditure Assessment (replaced by SSA)
GRIPP   Getting Research Into Purchasing and Practice
GSCC   General Social Care Council
GSI   Government Secure Intranet
GSL   General Sales List (a medicine which can be sold anywhere)
GSM   Global System of Mobility
GSOH   good sense of humour (as important in the health service as on the lonely hearts pages)
GSW   gunshot wound
GTAC   Gene Therapy Advisory Committee
GTLRC   Gypsy and Traveller Law Reform Coalition
GTN   Government Telephone Network
GUCH   Grown Up Congenital Heart Patients Association
GUI   graphical user interface
GUM   genito-urinary medicine (where STDs are treated)
GWC   General Whitley Council

H

H&S   health and safety
HA   health authority; housing association
HaCCRU   Health and Community Care Research Unit (based at Liverpool University)
HAG   Housing Association Grant
HAI   hospital-acquired infection
HARP   Hulme Action Research Project (works with people with mental health problems)
HAS   Health Advisory Service; human activity system
HASHD   hypertensive arteriosclerotic heart disease

HASSASSA   Health and Social Services and Social Security Adjudication Act

HAT   Housing Action Trust

HAWNHS   Health at Work in the NHS

HAZ   Health Action Zones (obsolete)

HB   Health Board (in Scotland); Housing Benefit

HBAI   households below average income

HBG   Health Benefit Group

HC   health circular; Healthcare Commission; Health Council; Huntingdon's chorea

HCA   historic cost accounting; Home Care Assistant (social care worker who provides domiciliary care; formerly known as home helps); Hospital Caterers Association

HCAG   Hospital Consultants Advisory Group (a steering body for projects on work patterns for consultants)

HCAI   healthcare associated infection

HCFA   Health Care Financing Administration (the federal agency that administers the Medicare, Medicaid and Child Health Insurance Programs in the US)

HCG   human chorionic gonadotrophin

HCHS   hospital and community health services (hospital services, ambulances and certain community health services such as district nursing; these services are provided mostly by NHS Trusts)

HCIA   Health Care Information (an American company which analyses health data; now part of Solucient)

HCS   Holiday Care Service

HCSP   Health Care Service for Prisoners

HCW   Health Care Worker (provides nursing support in clinical areas; NVQ qualified)

HDA   Health Development Agency (obsolete; now the National Institute for Health and Clinical Excellence [NICE]); Huntington's Disease Association

HDL   high-density lipoprotein

HDM   house dust mite

HDU   High Dependency Unit (one step down from the ITU)

HE   health education; higher education

HEA   Health Education Authority (now replaced by the HAD); Health Equity Audit

HEASIG   High Ethnicity Authorities' Special Issues Group

HEBS   Health Education Board for Scotland

HEED   Health Economic Evaluations Database
HEFC   Higher Education Funding Council
HEFCE   Higher Education Funding Council for England
HEFMA   Health Estates and Facilities Management Association
HEI   higher education institution
HEIF   Higher Education Innovation Fund
HELMIS   Health Management Information Service (Nuffield Institute, Leeds)
HEO   health education officer
HEP   Health Education Partnership
HEPA   high efficiency particulate air
HERO   Higher Education and Research Opportunities in the UK
HEROINE   Health Electronic Resources Online in Northern England
HES   Hospital Episode Statistics; Hospital Eye Service
HEVU   Health Education Video Unit
HFEA   Human Fertilisation and Embryology Authority
HfHT   Help for Health Trust (obsolete)
HFMA   Healthcare Financial Management Association
HGAC   Human Genetics Advisory Commission
HGC   Human Genetics Commission
HHT   hand-held terminal
HIA   health impact assessment; Housing Improvement Agency
HIBCC   Health Index Bar Code Council; Health Index Business Communications Council
HImP   Health Improvement Programme
HIP   Health Investment Programme
HIPE   Hospital In-Patient Enquiry Scheme
HIS   health service indicators
HIS   hospital information system
HISN   High Individual Support Needs
HISS   hospital information and support system
HIU   Health Inequalities Unit
HIV   human immunodeficiency virus
HIYE   Health in Your Environment
HJSC   Hospital Junior Staff Committee (of BMA)
HL7   Health Level 7 (a healthcare-specific communication standard for data exchange between computer applications)
HLC   Healthy Living Centre
HLF   Heritage Lottery Fund

HLI Healthy Living Initiative
HLPI high level performance indicator
HM HNA Health Needs Assessment
HMIC Health Management Information Consortium
HMO health maintenance organisation (US); house in multiple occupation
HMR hospital medical record
HMSO Her Majesty's Stationery Office (now TSO)
HNI Housing Needs Index
HO Home Office; House Officer
HoN Health of the Nation White Paper on Prevention
HoNOS Health of the Nation Outcomes Scale
HOWIS Health of Wales Information Service (the official website for NHS in Wales)
HP health promotion
HPA Health Protection Agency
HPC Health Professions Council
HPC Health Professions Council
HPE Health Promotion England (obsolete); higher professional education
HPERU Health Policy and Economic Research Unit
HPH health-promoting hospital
HPMA Healthcare People Management Association
HPR health process re-design
HPSS Health Promotion Specialist Service; Health and Personal Social Services
HPU Health Protection Unit
HR human resources (personnel)
HRD human resource development
HRD-MET Human Resources Directorate-Medical Education and Development
HRG Healthcare Resource Group
HRQOL health-related quality of life
HSAC Health Service Advisory Committee (of HSE)
HSC Health Select Committee; Health and Safety Commission; Health Service Circular (management letters from the DoH replacing ELs, HSGs, FDLs and FHSLs); Health Service Commissioner
HSCA Health and Social Care Authority (Northern Ireland)
HSCI Health Service Cost Index
HSCIC Health and Social Care Information Centre

HSCT   Health and Social Care Trust (Northern Ireland)
HSDU   hospital sterile and disinfection unit
HSE   Health and Safety Executive
HSG   health service guidance; Health Strategy Group; Housing Support Grant
HSJ   *Health Services Journal*
HSMC   Health Services Management Centre (University of Birmingham)
HSP   Healthy Schools Programme; heart sink patient
HSPI   Health Service Prices Index
HSPSCB   High Security Psychiatric Services Commissioning Board (obsolete)
HSSB   Health and Social Services Board (Northern Ireland)
HSSC   Health and Social Services Council (Northern Ireland)
HST   higher surgical trainee (a senior registrar in old speak); higher surgical training
HSTAT   Health Services/Technology Assessment Text
HSV   herpes simplex virus
HSW   health and safety at work
HSWA   Health and Safety at Work Act 1974
HTA   Health Technology Assessment; Human Tissue Authority
HTAI   Health Technology Assessment International
HTCS   Hospital Travel Cost Scheme
HTH   hope this helps
HTM   high technology medicine
HV   health visitor; home visit
HVA   Health Visitors Association
HVHSC   Human and Veterinary Healthcare Sectoral Consultation (bringing together interested bodies in the public and private sectors to draw up key principles concerning biotechnology and genetically modified organisms)
HWI   Healthy Workplace Initiative
HWRC   Household Waste Recycling Centre

I

I&D   incision and drainage
IADL   instrumental activities of daily living
IAG   information age government
IAGI   intended average gross income (of GPs) (the total money paid on average to GPs, i.e. inclusive of indirectly reimbursed expenses)

IAMRA International Association of Medical Regulatory Authorities

IANI intended average net income (of GPs) (the total money paid on average to GPs, exclusive of indirectly reimbursed expenses)

IANR intended average net remuneration

IAPO International Alliance of Patients' Organisations

IAVI International Aids Vaccine Initiative

IBD interest-bearing debt

IBMS Institute of Biomedical Science

IBNR incurred but not reported (clinical negligence liability)

IC Information Commissioner

ICA Invalid Care Allowance (now replaced by Carers Allowance)

ICAS Independent Complaints Advocacy Service

ICC Integrated Child Credit

ICD The WHO's International Statistical Classification of Diseases and Related Health Problems (now in its 10th revision)

ICE Intercollegiate Examination

ICES Institute for Clinical Evaluative Sciences

ICFM Institute of Charity Fundraising Managers Trust

ICHS International Centre for Health and Society

ICIDH International Classification of Impairment, Activities and Participation

ICN infection control nurse; integrated care network

ICP integrated care pathway; Integrated Care Pilots; intra-cranial pressure

ICRC International Committee of the Red Cross

ICRS Integrated Care Records Service

ICT infection control team; information communication technology

ICU intensive care unit

ICW Indigenous Community Worker; integrated clinical workstation

ICWS integrated clinical workstation

ID2000 Indices of Deprivation 2000

IDA Improvement Development Agency

IDDM insulin-dependent diabetes mellitus

IdeA Improvement and Development Agency

IDF International Diabetes Federation

IELTS International English Language Testing Service

IEMC Inter-Balkan European Medical Centre

I4H Information for Health
IFM Information for the Management of Healthcare
IFPMA International Federation of Pharmaceutical Manufacturers Associations
IFRS International Financial Reporting Standards
IG information governance
IGSoC Information Governance Statement of Compliance
IHA Independent Healthcare Association of 600 independent hospitals and homes
IHCD Institute of Health and Care Development
IHE Institute of Hospital Engineering; International Health Exchange
IHEEM Institute of Healthcare Engineering and Estate Management
IHF International Hospital Federation
IHM Institute of Healthcare Management
IHRIM Institute of Health Record Information and Management
IHSM Institute of Health Service Managers (now part of the IHM)
IIP Investors in People (initiative)
ILA Individual Learning Account
ILAF Independent Local Advisory Forum
ILCOR International Liaison Committee on Resuscitation
ILD Index of Local Deprivation (replaced by IMD)
ILF Independent Living Fund
ILP Independent Living Project
ILSI International Life Sciences Institute
IM&T information management and technology
IMA Irish Medical Association
IMC Information Management Centre
IMCA independent mental capacity advocate
IMD Index of Multiple Deprivations
IMG international medical graduates
IMGE Information Management Group of NHS Executive
IMHO in my humble opinion; in my honest opinion
IMLS Institute of Medical Laboratory Sciences
IMR infant mortality rate
INASP International Network for the Availability of Scientific Publications
INES International Network of Engineers and Scientists for Global Responsibility

INSET in-service training
IOP Institute of Psychiatry
IoS Item of Service (something that GPs get paid for on a itemised basis under the terms of the Red Book)
IP inpatient
IPF Institute of Public Finance
IPH Improvement Partnership for Hospitals
IPM Institute of Personnel Management
IPPC Integrated Pollution Prevention Control
IPPF International Planned Parenthood Federation
IPPR Institute for Public Policy Research
IPR independent professional review; individual performance review; intellectual property rights
IPS Indicative Prescribing Scheme; Integrated Personnel System
IPU Information Policy Unit (DoH)
IQI Indicators for Quality Improvement
IRIS interactive resource information system
IRL Initial Resource Limit
IRO industrial relations officer
IRP Independent Reconfiguration Panel
IRR internal rate of return
IS Income Support (formerly Supplementary Benefit, before that National Assistance, before that the Poor Law)
ISB Information Standards Board (NHS); Intercollegiate Speciality Examinations Board; Invest to Save Budget
ISBN International Standard Book Number
ISCAP Integrating Surgical Curriculum and Practice
ISCP Intercollegiate Surgical Curriculum Project
ISD Information and Statistics Division (Scotland)
ISDD Institute for the Study of Drug Dependence
ISDN Integrated Services Digital Network
ISE individualised sensory environment
ISG Information Services Group
ISIP Integrated Service Improvement Programme
ISO Infrastructure Support Organisation; International Organization for Standardization
ISPOR International Society for Pharmacoeconomics and Outcomes Research
ISQua International Society for Quality in Health Care
ISS International Sponsorship Scheme (formerly ODTS)
ISSM Institute of Sterile Services Management

IST Intensive Support Team
ISTAHC International Society of Technology Assessment in Health Care
ISTC independent sector treatment centres
IT information technology
ITC independent treatment centre
ITN invitation to negotiate
ITS Independent Tribunal Service (now replaced by the Appeals Service)
ITT invitation to tender
ITU intensive therapy/treatment unit
IUHPE International Union for Health Promotion and Education
IV independent variable; intravenous
IWL Improving Working Lives
IYF inter-year flexibility

J

J judge (in law reports)
JAMA *Journal of the American Medical Association*
JANET Joint Academic Network
JCB Joint Commissioning Board
JCC Joint Consultative Committee; Joint Consultants Committee
JCCO Joint Council for Clinical Oncology
JCE Joint Commissioning Executive
JCHMT Joint Committee for Higher Medical Training
JCHST Joint Committee for Higher Surgical Training
JCPTGP Joint Committee on Postgraduate Training in General Practice
JCVI Joint Committee on Vaccination and Immunisation
JDC Junior Doctors Committee
JE job evaluation
JEMS *Journal of Emergency Medicine*
JEWP Job Evaluation Working Party
JFC Joint Formulary Committee
JFSSG Joint Food Safety and Standards Group
JHU Joint Health Unit
JIF Joint Investment Fund (Scotland)
JIGSAW project designed to reduce the need for hospital beds; co-ordinated by GMAS
JIP Joint Investment Plan (what you have to write in your BSVP group)

JISC Joint Information Systems Committee

JIT just in time (supplies delivery)

JLDS Joint Learning Disability Service (runs CLDTs)

JNC(J) Joint Negotiating Committee (on junior doctors terms and conditions of service)

JPAC Joint Planning Advisory Committee (replaced by SWAG)

JRCT Joseph Rowntree Charitable Trust

JRF Joseph Rowntree Foundation

JRG Joint Review Group

JSA Job Seeker's Allowance

JSE Joint Strategy Executive

JSG Joint Strategy Group

JSOG Joint Senior Officers Group

K

KED Kendrick extrication device

KF King's Fund

KFOA King's Fund Organisational Audit

KI key indicator (social services)

KIGS key indicators, geographical system

KISS keep it simple stupid

KSF Knowledge and Skills Framework (part of Agenda for Change)

KTD Kendrick traction device

KTP Knowledge Transfer Partnership

KVO keep veins open

L

LA local authority

LAA Local Area Agreement; Local Authority Association

LAC Local Authority Circular; Local Authority Company; looked after children

LACOTS Local Authorities Co-ordinating Body on Food and Trading Standards

LAD Local Authority District

LAF Local Advisory Forum

LAFS Local Authority Financial Settlement

LAG local advisory group

LAL local authority letter

LAN local area network

LAP local area partnership; local action plan

LAPIS   Locality and Practice Information System
LARIA   Local Authorities Research and Intelligence Association
LAS   Locum Appointment Service; London Ambulance Service
LASA   London Advice Services Alliance
LASFE   Local Authorities' Self-Financed Expenditure
LASS   Local Authority Social Services
LASSL   Local Authority Social Services Letter
LAT   locum appointment for training
LATF   Local Asthma Taskforce
LATS   London Academic Training Scheme (part of LIZEI)
LAWDC   Local Authority Waste Disposal Company
LCFS   Local Counter Fraud Specialist
LCMG   local communications user group
LD   learning difficulties; Liberal Democrat; local democracy
LD/MH   learning difficulties/mental handicap
LDA   Local Development Agency; London Development Agency
LDAF   Learning Disabilities Award Framework
LDC   Local Dental Committee (the statutory body of GDPs that represents dental practices in the local area)
LDP   Local Delivery Plan
LDSAG   Local Diabetes Service Advisory Group
LEA   Local Education Authority
LEC   Local Enterprise Company
LEI   Local Employment Initiative
LEL   lower explosive limit
LEO   Leading Empowered Organisations
LETS   Local Exchange Trading Scheme
LFS   Labour Force Survey
LGA   Local Government Association
LGBT   lesbian, gay, bisexual and transgender
LGC   Local Government Chronicle
LGFR   Local Government Finance Report
LGFS   Local Government Financial Settlement; Local Government Financial Statistics
LGHA   Local Government & Housing Act 1989
LGIB   Local Government International Bureau
LGIU   Local Government Information Unit
LGMB   Local Government Management Board
LGPS   Local Government Pension Scheme
LHB   local health boards (Wales)
LHC   Local Health Council

LHCC   Local Health Care Co-operative (Scottish variety of PCG)

LHG   Local Health Group (a sort of Welsh PCG)

LHP   Local Health Plan

LHSCG   Local Health and Social Carte Group (Northern Ireland)

LIF   Local Initiatives Fund

LIFT   Local Improvement Finance Trust

LIG   local implementation group

LIMS   laboratory information management systems

LINC   Library and Information Commission (obsolete)

LINks   Local Involvement Networks

LIO   Local Implementation Officer; Local Infrastructure Organisation

LIP   Local Implementation Plans

LIS   library information system; Local Implementation Strategy

LISI   Low Income Scheme Index (measure of deprivation based on claims for exemption from prescription charges on grounds of low income)

LIT   Local Implementation Team

LIZ   London Initiative Zone

LIZEI   London Implementation Zone Education Initiative

LLL   lifelong learning

LLSC   Local Learning and Skills Council

LLTI   limiting long-term illness

LMC   Local Medical Committee (statutory local committee for all GPs in the area covered by the health authority)

LMCA   Long-term Medical Conditions Alliance

LMWAG   Local Medical Workforce Advisory Groups (formed in 1996 to co-ordinate postgraduate medical education between groups of trusts; there are five or six in each NHS Region)

LNC   Local Negotiating Committee

LNRS   Local Neighbourhood Renewal Strategy

LOBNH   lights on but nobody home

LOS   length of stay (a measure of activity in hospital wards)

LPC   Local Pharmaceutical Committee (a committee of pharmacists)

LPfIT   London Programme for IT

LPI   labour productivity index

LPM   litres per minute

LPS   Local Pharmaceutical Services

LPSA   Local Public Service Agreement

LR   legitimate relationship

LRD Labour Research Department
LREC Local Research Ethics Committee
LRR Local Reference Rent
LRS Local and Regional Services
LSC Learning & Skills Council; Legal Services Commission
LSCG Local Specialised Commissioning Group
LSCS lower segment Caesarean section
LSHTM London School of Hygiene and Tropical Medicine
LSP local service provider(s); local strategic partnership
LSVT Large Scale Voluntary Transfer
LTA long-term agreement
LTC long-term condition
LTM Learning to Manage Health Information
LTP Local Transport Plan
LTPS Liability to Third Parties Scheme
LTSA long-term service agreement
LTVS long-term ventilatory support
LURG local user representative group
LWPG Local Winter Planning Group
LYS life years saved

M

MA Maternity Allowance
MAA Medical Artists Association of Great Britain
MAAG Medical Audit Advisory Group; Multi-disciplinary Audit Advisory Group
MAAQ Multidisciplinary Audit and Quality Group (replaced by the ACTS)
MAB Metropolitan Asylums Board (obsolete)
MAC Medical Advisory Committee
MACA Mental After Care Association
MADEL Medical and Dental Education Levy
MADEN Medical and Dental Education Network
MAF Management Accountancy Framework
MAGGOT medically able, go get other transportation
MALDA Multi-agency Learning Disability Assessment
MANCAS Manchester Care Assessment Schedule
MAP management action plan
MaPSaF Manchester Patient Safety Framework
MAR2C Matching Resources to Care (a mental health information system for caseload monitoring devised to study cases of serious

mental illness; IT can compare data from Social Services, Health Services and the voluntary sector)

MARMAP Multi-agency Risk Management Assessment Process

MARP Multi-agency Risk Assessment Panel (decides whether mentally ill people are dangerous)

MAS minimal access surgery

MASC Medical Academic Staff Committee; Medical Advisors Support Centre

MAST Multi-agency Support Team

MASTA Medical Advisory Services for Travellers Abroad

MAT Medical Appeal Tribunal

MAVIS Mobility Advice and Vehicle Information Service

MBA Master of Business Administration

MBTI Myers-Briggs Type Indicator (Myers-Briggs Personality Type Inventory)

MC Medicines Commission

MCA Medicines Control Agency; motorcycle accident

MCCD Medical Certificate of Cause of Death

MCI mass casualty incident

MCN managed clinical network

MCO managed care organisation

MCP male chauvinist pig (obsolete?); medical care practitioner

MCRG Medical Career Research Group

MCSP Member of the Chartered Society of Physiotherapy

MDA Medical Devices Agency

MDAP Multi-Deanery Appointment Process

MDD Medical Devices Directorate

MDDUS Medical and Dental Defence Union of Scotland

MDG Management Development Group (Scotland); Muscular Dystrophy Group

MDI metered dose inhaler

MDM medical decision making

MDO mentally disordered offender

MDR multiple drug resistant

MDS minimum data set

MDT mobile data terminal; multi-disciplinary team

MDU Medical Defence Union

ME Management Executive

MEC Management Education for Clinicians; Management Executive Committee

MEDITEL GP information system

MEDLARS Medical Literature Analysis and Retrieval System
MEDS Medical Deputising Service
MEE Medical Education for England
MEL Management Executive Letter (Scotland)
MENCAP Royal Society for Mentally Handicapped Children and Adults
MEQ modified examination question
MeReC bulletin published by the National Prescribing Centre on evidence based therapeutics
MERV Medical Emergency Response Vehicle
MESB Medical Education Standards Board
MeSH Medical Subject Headings
MESOL Management Education Scheme by Open Learning
MFF market forces factor
MFS market forces supplement
MGA Myasthenia Gravis Association
MGRG Management Guidance Review Group
MHA Mental Health Act 1983
MHAC Mental Health Act Commission
MHC major histocompatability complex
MHE Mental Health Enquiry
MHG Mental Health Grant
MHIG Mental Health Information Group
MHIS Mental Health Information Strategy
MHMDS Mental Health Minimum Data Set
MHPAF Mental Health Performance Assessment Framework
MHPSS Manchester Health Promotion Specialist Service
MHRA Medicines and Healthcare Products Regulatory Agency
MHRT Mental Health Review Tribunal (convened to hear appeals against detention under the MHA)
MHT Mental Health Task Force
MIA Medical Insurance Agency
MIDIRS Midwife Information and Resource Service
MIE Medical Informatics Europe
MIG Medical Information Group
MIMMS Major Incident Medical Management and Support
MIMS Monthly Index of Medical Specialties
MINAP Myocardial Infarction National Audit Project
MIND organisation of mental health users
MINI Mental Illness Needs Index
Mini-CEX Mini Clinical Evaluation Exercise

Mini-PAT   Peer Assessment Tool (360-degree)
Mini-PBA   Procedure-based Assessment (single procedure)
MIQUEST   A method of extracting information from GP computer systems
MIS   management information systems
MISG   Mental Illness Specific Grant (government subsidy to supplement spending by local authorities on social care for mentally ill people living in the community)
MIT   Massachusetts Institute of Technology; minimally invasive therapy
MITAG   Medical Information and Technology Advisory Group
MIU   minor injuries unit
MLA   medical laboratory assistant; Museums, Libraries and Archives Council
MLA   Member of the Legislative Assembly (Northern Ireland)
MLCF   Medical Leadership Competency Framework
MLD   mild learning disability
MLSO   Medical Laboratory Scientific Officer
MMC   Modernising Medical Careers
MMR   measles, mumps, rubella
MMS   Medical Management Services
MMSAC   Medical Manpower Standing Advisory Committee (representatives from BMA, Royal Colleges, Regional Manpower committees, Medical Research Council and Council of Deans)
MNC   Modernising Nursing Careers
MO   Medical Officer
MOD   Ministry of Defence
MOH   Medical Officer of Health (a predecessor of the DPH)
MOI   mechanism of injury
MOP   Mobile Optical Practice
MOR   Millennium Operating Regime
MoU   memorandum of understanding
MPA   Masters in Public Administration; Medical Prescribing Adviser
MPC   Medical Practices Committee (abolished 2002)
MPDS   Medical Priority Dispatch System
MPET   Multi-professional Education and Training levy
MPIG   minimum practice income guarantee
MPS   Medical Protection Society; Modernising Public Services Group

MPT maximum part time
MPU Medical Practitioners Union
MRC Medical Research Council
MREC Multi-centre Research Ethics Committee
MRFIT Multiple Risk Factor Intervention Trial
MRI magnetic resonance imaging
MRO Medical Records Officer
MRP Minimum Revenue Provision (part of capital control framework)
MRSA methicillin-resistant *Staphylococcus aureus*
MSAC Maternity Services Advisory Committee
MSD Merck Sharp & Dohme Ltd
MSDS Material Safety Data Sheet
MSEB Medical Standards Education Board (replacing JCPTGP and STA)
MSF union for skilled and professional workers, including many NHS employees (formerly ASTMS, now joined into AMICUS; Medicine Sans Frontières; multi-source feedback)
MSGP-4 National Study of Morbidity in General Practice
MSI Marie Stopes International
MSLC Maternity Services Liaison Committee (brings together professions involved in maternity services with laypeople to agree procedures and monitor their effectiveness as they appear to individual women)
MSP Member of the Scottish Parliament
MSPCG Most Sparsely Populated Councils Group
MSU medium secure unit; short for MSSU
MTA Management Team Assistant
MTAS Medical Training Application Service
MTFP Medium Term Financial Plan
MTO Medical Technical Officer
MUSCLE Multi-Station Clinical Examination
MV Millennium Volunteer
MWC Mental Welfare Commission
MWCS Mental Welfare Commission for Scotland
MWEP Medical Workforce Expansion Programme
MWF Women's Medical Federation
MWSAC Medical Workforce Standing Advisory Committee (working for the education committee of the GMC on appraising doctors and dentists in training for SCOPME

and on general clinical training during the pre-registration year)

MWSAG Medical Workforce Standing Advisory Group

N

N3 New National Network (Broadband)
N&MC Nursing and Midwifery Council
NA Nursing Auxiliary
NAAS National Association of Air Ambulance Services
NAB National Assistance Board (1948–66)
NAC National Abortion Campaign
NACAB National Association of Citizens Advice Bureaux
NACC National Association for Colitis and Crohn's Disease
NACEPD National Advisory Council on Employment of People with Disabilities
NACGP National Association of Commissioning GPs
NACPME National Advice Centre for Postgraduate Medical Education
NACRO National Association for the Care and Resettlement of Offenders
NACT National Association of Clinical Tutors
NACVS National Association of Councils for Voluntary Service
NAFHP National Association of Fundholding Practices (obsolete)
NAGPT National Association of GP Tutors
NAGS NICE Appraisal Groups
NAGST National Advisory Group for Scientists and Technicians
NAHAT National Association of Health Authorities and Trusts (obsolete)
NAHCSM National Association of Health Care Supplies Managers
NAHSSO National Association of Health Service Security Officers
NAHWT National Association of Health Workers and Travellers
NALHF National Association of Leagues of Hospital Friends
NANOS North American Neuro-Opthalmology Society
NANP National Association of Non-Principals (now NASGP)
NANT National Appraisal of New Technologies
NAO National Audit Office
NAPC National Association of Primary Care (formed from the embers of Fundholding National Association to represent interests of PCGs)
NAPMECA National Association of Postgraduate Medical Education Centre Administration

NAPP   National Association for Patient Participation
NAPS   National Anti-Poverty Strategy (Ireland)
NAS   National Autistic Society
NASEN   National Association for Special Educational Needs
NASGP   National Association of Sessional GPs (representing Locums, Freelance GPs and Salaried GPs, i.e. Non Principals)
NASP   National Application Service Provider
NASS   National Asylum Support Service
NATN   National Association of Theatre Nurses; National Association of Training Nurses
NatPaCT   National Primary and Care Trust (development programme)
NAVB   National Association of Volunteer Bureaux
NAVHO   National Association of Voluntary Help Organisations
NAW   National Assembly for Wales
NAWO   National Alliance of Women's Organisations
NBA   National Blood Authority (England)
NBAP   National Booked Admissions Programme
NBG   lacking evidence of effectiveness
NBI   National Beds Inquiry
NBS   National Board for Nursing, Midwifery and Health Visiting for Scotland (obsolete)
NBTS   National Blood Transfusion Service (obsolete)
NBV   net book value
NCAA   National Clinical Assessment Authority
NCAS   National Clinical Assessment Service (formerly NCAA National Clinical Assessment Authority)
NCASP   National Clinical Audit Support Programme
NCBV   National Coalition for Black Volunteering
NCC   National Consumer Council
NCCA   National Centre for Clinical Audit (now absorbed into NICE); National Community Care Alliance
NCCG   Non-Consultant Career Grade
NCCHTA   National Co-ordinating Centre for Health Technology Assessment
NCCSDO   National Co-ordinating Centre for NHS Service Delivery and Organisation Research and Development (at the London School of Hygiene and Tropical Medicine)
NCE   National Confidential Enquiry; net current expenditure
NCEPOD   National Confidential Enquiry into Patient Outcome and Death (formerly CEPOD)

NCG National Commissioning Group
NCH National Children's Home, now known as Action For Children
NCI National Captioning Institute
NCI National Confidential Inquiry; NHS Centre for Involvement
NCIL National Centre for Independent Living
NCIS National Criminal Intelligence Service
NCISH National Confidential Inquiry into Suicide and Homicide by people with Mental Illness
NCL National Civic League
NCMO National Casemix Office
NCSC National Care Standards Commission (abolished 2004)
NCSSD National Counselling Service for Sick Doctors
NCT National Childbirth Trust
NCV National Centre for Volunteering (obsolete)
NCVCCO National Council of Voluntary Child Care Organisations
NCVO National Council for Voluntary Organisations
NCVQ National Council for Vocational Qualifications
NCVYS National Council for Voluntary Youth Services
ND New Deal
NDC National Disability Council; New Deal for Communities
NDPB non-departmental public body
NDPHS National Disabled Persons Housing Service
NDT National Development Team for People with Learning Disabilities
NDTMS National Drug Treatment Monitoring System
NDU Nurse Development Unit
NDYP New Deal for Young People
NEAT new and emerging applications of technology
NED non-executive director
NEET not in education, employment or training
NEJM *New England Journal of Medicine*
NeLH National Electronic Library for Health
NERC Natural Environment Research Council
NES NHS Education for Scotland
NESTA National Endowment for Science Technology and the Arts
NET new and emerging technologies
NF Nuffield Foundation
NFA no fixed address
NFAP National Framework for Assessing Performance

NFI   National Fraud Initiative
NFP   not-for-profit
NFR   not for resuscitation
NFW   no further work
NGfL   National Grid for Learning
nGMS   New General Medical Services (contract)
NGO   non-governmental organisation
NHAIS   National Health Authority Information Systems
NHD   notional half day (consultants)
NHF   National Heart Forum
NHFA   Nursing Homes Fees Agency
NHIS   National Health Intelligence Service
NHLI   National Heart and Lung Institute, Imperial College
NHS CFH   NHS Connecting for Health
NHS CRS   NHS Care Records Service
NHS EED   NHS Economic Evaluation Database
NHS EHU   NHS Ethnical Health Unit
NHS FAM   NHS Fraud Awareness Month
NHS IMC   NHS Information Centre
NHS KSF   NHS Knowledge and Skills Framework
NHS LIFT   NHS Local Improvement Finance Trust
NHS PSA   NHS Purchasing and Supply Agency
NHS QIS   NHS Quality Improvement Scotland
NHS   National Health Service
NHS(S)   National Health Service in Scotland
NHS/N3   replaced the private NHS communications network NHSnet
NHSAC   National Health Service Appointments Commission
NHSAR   National Health Service Administrative Register
NHSBSA   NHS Business Services Authority
NHSBSP   NHS Breast Screening Programme
NHSCA   NHS Consultants Association
NHSCCA   NHS and Community Care Act (1990)
NHSCCC   NHS Centre for Coding and Classification
NHSCR   NHS Central Register
NHSCSF   NHS Counter Fraud Service
NHSCSFMS   NHS Counter Fraud and Security Management Service
NHSCTA   NHS Clinical Trials Adviser
NHSE   NHS Estates; NHS Executive (abolished 2002)
NHSFT   NHS Foundation Trust

NHSI NHS Institute for Innovation and Improvement
NHSIA NHS Information Authority (abolished 2005)
NHSIII NHS Institute for Innovation and Improvement
NHSL NHS Logistics
NHSLA NHS Litigation Authority
NHSmail NHS email and directory service
NHSME National Health Service Management Executive (Scotland)
NHSME NHS Management Executive (in England; now called the NHSE)
NHSMEE NHS Medical Education England
NHSnet Intranet for the NHS
NHSOE NHS Overseas Enterprises
NHSP NHS Partners
NHSPA NHS Pensions Agency (now merged as part of the NHS Business Services Authority, NHSBSA)
NHSPA NHS Pensions Authority
NHSS NHS Scotland; NHS Supplies; National Healthy Schools Standard
NHSSMS NHS Security Management Service
NHST NHS Trust
NHSTD NHS Training Directorate; NHS Training Division
NHSTF NHS Trust Federation
NHSTU NHS Training Unit
NHSU National Health Service University (obsolete)
NI National Insurance
NIA Northern Ireland Assembly
NIACE National Institute of Adult and Continuing Education
NIAS Northern Ireland Ambulance Service
NIC National Insurance Contribution; net ingredient cost (the basic price of a drug)
NICARE Northern Ireland Centre for Health Care Co-operation and Development
NICE National Institute for Clinical Excellence; National Institute for Health and Clinical Excellence; Northern Institute for Continuing Education
NICEC National Institute for Carers and Educational Counselling
NICON NHS Confederation in Northern Ireland
NICS Northern Ireland Civil Service
NICU Neonatal Intensive Care Unit
NICVA Northern Ireland Council for Voluntary Action

NIH National Institute of Health; Nuffield Institute for Health (Leeds)

NIHR National Institute for Health Research

NIHSS Nosocomial Infection National Surveillance Scheme

NILO National Investment and Loans Office

NIMHE National Institute for Mental Health in England

NINo National Insurance Number

NISW National Institute of Social Work (obsolete)

NJC National Joint Council

NLC (DoH) National Leadership Council

NLDB National Leadership Development Bodies

NLH National Library for Health

NLIAH National Leadership and Innovation Agency for Healthcare (Wales)

NLM National Library of Medicine

NLN The National Leadership Network for Health and Social Care

NLOP NPfIT Local Ownership Programme

NMAC National Medical Advisory Committee

NMAP Nursing Midwifery and Allied Health Professionals (Internet resource)

NMC Nursing and Midwifery Council

NMDS nursing minimum data set

NMEfIT North, Midlands and East Programme for IT

NMET Non-medical Education and Training

NMIS Nurse Management Information System

NMS National Minimum Standards

NNH number needed to harm

NNT number needed to treat

NOF National Opportunities Fund

NOMDS National Organ Matching and Distribution Service (*see* UHTSSA)

NOMIS National Online Manpower Information Service

NOP National Opinion Polls

NOS National Occupation Standards

NP Non-Principal

NPA National Pharmaceutical Association

NPAT National Patients' Access Team

NPC National Prescribing Centre (based in Liverpool; formerly known as MASC; publishes *MeReC Bulletin* which is distributed to all GPs on request); net present cost

NPCRDC National Primary Care Research and Development Centre (based in the University of Manchester)
NPfIT National Programme for IT (in the NHS)
NPG Modernising Health and Social Services: National Priorities Guidance
NPHS National Public Health Service (Wales)
NPHT Nuffield Provincial Hospitals Trust
NPIS National Poisons Information Service
NPL National Physical Laboratory
NPN National PALS Network
NPRB Nurses Pay Review Body
NPSA National Patient Safety Agency
NPT near patient testing
NPV net present value
NR nearest relative
NRAC NHS Scotland Resource Allocation Committee
NRC National Regionalisation Consortium
NRCI national reference cost index
NRE non-recurring expenditure
NRES National Research Ethics Service
NRLS National Reporting and Learning Service
NRPB National Radiological Protection Board
NRR National Research Register
NRS Neighbourhood Renewal Strategy
NRT nicotine replacement therapy
NSC National Screening Committee (UK)
NSCAG National Specialist Commissioning Advisory Group (succeeded by The National Commissioning Group, NCG)
NSCG The National Specialised Commissioning Group
NSEC National Smoking Education Campaign
NSF National Schizophrenia Fellowship (now called Rethink); National Service Framework; National Stakeholder Forum
NSFMH National Service Framework – Mental Health
NSMI National Sports Medicine Institute (UK)
NSPCC National Society for the Prevention of Cruelty to Children
NSRC National Schedule of Reference Costs
NSS National Services Scotland
NSTS NHS Strategic Tracing Service
NSU non-specific urethritis (common STD)
NSV National Supplies Vocabulary
NTA National Treatment Agency

NTAC   NHS Technology Adoption Centre
NTN   National Training Number
NTO   National Training Organisation
NTT   nuchal translucency thickness (screening method for Down's syndrome)
NTTRL   National Tissue Typing Reference Laboratory
NVP   newly vulnerable person
NVQ   National Vocational Qualification
NWCS   Nation Wide Clearing Service (all trusts must submit data about admitted patient care which is then forwarded to HAs)
NWIPP   National Workforce Information and Planning Programme
NWN   NHS-wide networking
NWSI   Nurse with a Special Interest
NYCDOHMH   New York City Department of Health and Mental Hygiene

O

O&M   organisation and methods
OAPS   Objective Assessment of Professional Skills
OAT   Out of Area Treatment (the replacement for ECR)
OBC   outline business case
OBD   occupied bed day
OBS   output based specification
OCD   obsessive compulsive disorder
OCMO   Office of the Chief Medical Officer (Wales)
OCN   Open College Network
OCPA   Office of the Commissioner for Public Appointments
OCR   optical character reader; optical character recognition
OCS   order communication system; Organisational Codes Service
OD   once daily; organisational development; outside diameter; overdose
ODA   Operating Department assistant; Overseas Development Agency; Overseas Doctors Agency
ODO   Operating Department orderly
ODP   Operating Department practitioner
ODPM   Office of the Deputy Prime Minister
ODTS   Overseas Doctors Training Scheme (of appropriate Royal College)

OECD Organisation for Economic Co-operation and Development

OEL occupational exposure limit

Ofsted Office for Standards in Education

OGC Office for Government Commerce

OH occupational health

OHAG Oral Health Advisory Group

OHE Office of Health Economics (London)

OHN *Our Healthier Nation* (Cm3852, www.ohn.gov.uk)

OHS Occupational Health Service

OIC Officer in Charge

OIE Office International des Epizooties

OIHCP Office for Information on Health Care Performance

OISC Office of the Immigration Services Commissioner

OJEC *Official Journal of the European Community*

OME Office of Manpower Economics

OMNI Organising Medical Networked Information

OMP Ophthalmic Medical Practitioner

OMV open market value

OMVEU open market value in existing use

ONS Office for National Statistics (the result of a merger in April 1996 of the Central Statistical Office and the Office of Population Censuses and Surveys)

OO optometrist

OOH out of hours

OOP Out of Programme

OOPC Out of Programme for career break

OOPE Out of Programme for experience

OOPR Out of Programme for research

OOPT Out of Programme for clinical training

OP outpatient

OPAC Online Public Access Catalogue

OPCS Office of Population, Census and Surveys (system for classifying disease and treatment; now Office for National Statistics, ONS)

OPD Outpatient Department

OPHIS Office for Public Health in Scotland

OPM Office of Public Management

OR operation research (a scientific method which uses models of a system to evaluate alternative courses of action with a view to improving decision making)

OSB Other Services Block (now replaced by EPCS)
OSC Overview and Scrutiny Committee (local authority)
OSCE Observed Structured Clinical Examination
OSCHR Office for the Strategic Coordination of Health Research
OSDLS Open Source Digital Library System
OST Office of Science and Technology
OT occupational therapist; occupational therapy
OTC over the counter (medicines not requiring a prescription)
OU Open University
OVE occlusive vascular event
OWAM Organisation with a Memory
OWW One World Week
OXERA Oxford Economic Research Associates

P

P&T professional and technical
PA Patients Association (patient's mechanism to communicate
with medical services); personal assistant; physician assistant
(US); Police Authority
PABX Public Area Branch Exchange
PAC Public Accounts Committee
PACE Police & Criminal Evidence Act 1984; Promoting Action
on Clinical Effectiveness; Property Advisers to the Civil Estate
PACS Picture Archiving and Communication System
PACT Placing, Assessment and Counselling Team; Prescribing
Analysis and Costs (GPs get regular PACT reports from the
PPA giving details of their recent prescribing, comparing them
with local and national averages)
PAD peripheral arterial disease
PAF Performance Assessment Framework; Public Audit Forum
PAGB Proprietary Association of Great Britain
PALS Patient Advice and Liaison Service
PAMIS Parliamentary Monitoring and Intelligence Service
PAMP pathogen associated molecular pattern
PAMs professions allied to medicine (physiotherapists,
occupational therapists, etc.)
PAR programme analysis and review
PARN Professional Associations Research Network
PAS Patient Administration System (a main hospital database);
physician-assisted suicide
PASA Purchasing and Supply Agency

PASG pneumatic anti-shock garment

PAT Personnel Accountability Tag; Policy Action Team

PAYE pay as you earn

PBA Procedure Based Assessment (may be in parts; *see* Mini-PBA)

PBC practice-based commissioning; Public Benefit Corporation

PBL problem-based learning

PBMA programme budgeting and marginal analysis

PbR payment by results

PBR Pre-Budget Report

PBRS Public Benefit Recording System

PBx Private Branch Exchange (type of internal telephone network)

PC Patients' Council; Parish Council; personal computer; politically correct; primary care; public convenience

PCA patient controlled analgesia (usually a morphine pump)

PCAG Primary Care Audit Group (i.e. multi-disciplinary)

PCAPs Primary Care Act Pilots (the NHS (Primary Care) Act 1997 allowed NHS Trusts, NHS employees, qualified bodies and suitably experienced medical practitioners to submit proposals to provide general medical services under a contract with the health authority)

PCC primary care centre

PCG Primary Care Group (obsolete, *see* HSC 1998/230)

PCHR Personal Child Health Record

PCIP Primary Care Investment Plan

PCL Provision for Credit Liabilities

PCMCN Peninsula Cardiac Managed Clinical Network

PCO primary care organisation (generic term for PCT in England, Health and Social Services Board in Northern Ireland, Local Health Board in Wales and Primary Care Division within Area Health Board in Scotland)

PCP person-centred planning; personal communication profile

PCRC Primary Care Resource Centre

PCRTA Primary Care Research Team Assessment

PCS Public and Commercial Services Union

PCS/E Patient Classification System/Europe

PCT primary care trust

PDC public dividend capital (a form of long-term government finance on which the NHS trust pays dividends to the government. PDC has no fixed remuneration or repayment obligations, but in the long term the overall return on PDC is expected to be no less than on an equivalent loan)

PDD pervasive development disorder; prescribed daily dose (the average daily dose which is actually prescribed)

PDF Partnership Development Fund

PDO property damage only

PDP personal development plan; practice development plan

PDR Personal Development Review

PDS Parkinson's Disease Society; Personal Demographics Service; Personal Dental Services

PDSA plan, do, study, act

PE physical examination; pulmonary embolism

PEA pulseless electrical activity

PEAT Patient Environment Action Team

PEC Professional Executive Committee

PECS Picture Exchange Communication System

PEDC Potential Elderly Domiciliary Clients (part of SSA)

PEDW Patient Episode Database Wales

PEG percutaneous endoscopic gastrostomy

PEM prescription event monitoring

PES Public Expenditure Survey

PESC Public Expenditure Survey Committee (obsolete)

PESR Potential Elderly Supported Residents (part of SSA)

PET positron emission tomography

PETA People for the Ethical Treatment of Animals

PETS Paediatric Emergency Transfer Service

PEWP Public Expenditure White Paper

PF Patients' Forum

PFC patient-focused care; Professional Fees Committee

PFI Private Finance Initiative (now replaced by PPP)

PfIT Programmes for IT

PFMA Practice Fund Management Allowance (Allowance given to GP fundholders to manage their allocation. The allowance is primarily spent upon staff and equipment.)

PFU Private Finance Unit

PGCME Postgraduate and Continuing Medical Education

PGD Patient Group Directions; Postgraduate Dean

PGEA Postgraduate Education Allowance

PGMDE Postgraduate Medical and Dental Education

PGY3 Postgraduate Year 3 (= ST1)

PHA Public Health Alliance (now part of UKPHA)

PHAB physically disabled and able-bodied
PHANYC Public Health Association of New York City
PHC primary healthcare
PHCDS public health common data set
PHCSG Primary Health Care Specialist Group
PHCT Primary Health Care Team
PHeL Public Health Electronic Library
PHIS Public Health Institute of Scotland
PHL Public Health Laboratory
PHLS Public Health Laboratory Service
PHO Public Health Observatory
PHOENIX Primary Healthcare Organisations Exchanging New
  Ideas for Excellence
PHP public health practitioner
PHPU Public Health Policy Unit
PHRRC Public Health Research and Resource Centre (at the
  University of Salford)
PHSS Personal Health Summary System
PI parallel imports; performance indicator
PIA Partnership in Action; patient impact assessment; personal
  injury accident
PICKUP Professional, Industrial and Commercial Updating
PICS Platform for Internet Content Selection
PICU Paediatric ICU; Psychiatric ICU
PIDA Public Interest Disclosure Act
PIF Patient Information Forum
PIG Policy Implementation Groups; professional interest group;
  Promoting Independence Grant
PIL patient information leaflet
PIMS product information management system
PIN personal identification number; prior identification notice
PIU Performance and Innovation Unit
PLAB Professional and Linguistic Assessment Board
PLICS patient-led information and costing systems
PLP personal learning plan
PLPI Product Licence Parallel Import
PLT Protected Learning Time
PM project management
PMA Personal Medical Attendant (what insurance companies etc.
  call a doctor who writes a report for them)
PMCPA Prescription Medicines Code of Practice Authority

PMD Performance Management Directorate
PMD Prescribing Monitoring Document
PMETB Postgraduate Medical Education and Training Board
PMF Performance Management Framework
PMI private medical insurance
PMLD Profound and Multiple Learning Disabilities
PMR physical medicine and rehabilitation; progressive muscle relaxation
PMS personal medical service; post marketing surveillance; Primary Medical Services Contract
PND post-natal depression
PNL Prior Notification List (of patients for screening)
POC point of care
POCT point of care testing
PODS patient's own drugs
POINT Publications on the Internet (Department of Health)
POISE Procurement of Information Systems Effectively (The standard procedure followed for procurement of information systems.)
POLIS Parliamentary Online Indexing Service
POLST Physicians Orders for Life Sustaining Treatment
POM prescription-only medicine
POMR problem-oriented medical records
POPPs Partnerships for Older People Projects
POPUMET Protection of Persons Undergoing Medical Examination (regulations)
POSIX Portable Operating System Interface
POU Pulmonary Oncology Unit (chest cancers)
POVA Protection of Vulnerable Adults from Abuse
PPA Prescription Pricing Authority (costed all prescriptions dispensed in England in order to pay chemists for the costs of the drugs etc. they dispense; now done by NHSBSA)
PPBS Planning, Programming & Budgeting System
PPC promoting patient choice
PPDP Practice Professional Development Plans
PPDR Practice Profession Development and Revalidation
PPE personal protective equipment
PPF Priorities and Planning Framework
PPG Planning Policy Guidance; Principal Police Grant
PPI Patient and public involvement; proton pump inhibitor
PPIF Patient and public involvement forum (replaced by LINks)

PPM   planned preventative maintenance
PPO   preferred provider organisation
PPP   Private Patients Plan; public private partnership
PPPFC   Private Practice and Professionals Fees Committee
PPPP   Public-Private Partnership Programme (aka 4Ps)
PPRD   programme for provisionally registered doctors
PPRS   Pharmaceutical Price Regulation Scheme
PPU   Private Patients Unit
PQ   parliamentary question; post qualification
PQASSO   Practical Quality Assurance System for Small
   Organisations
PR   per rectum; public relations (no known connection?)
PRA   preventing and responding to aggression
PRB   Pay Review Body
PREPP   Post Registration Education and Preparation for Practice
   (nurses)
PRHO   Pre-Registration House Officer
PRIAE   Policy Research Institute on Ageing and Ethnicity
PRIMIS   Primary Care Information Services
PRINCE   Projects in Controlled Environments (a standard project
   management methodology used in all NHS Information
   systems projects)
PRO   Public Record Office
PRODIGY   Prescribing RatiOnally with Decision-support In
   General-practice studY
PRP   performance-related pay
PRT   personal risk training
PRU   Police Resources Unit (part of Home Office)
PSA   prostate-specific antigen; public service agreement
PSBR   Public Sector Borrowing Requirement
PSC   Public Sector Comparator
PSFD   Public Sector Financing Deficit
PSG   Prescribing Strategy Group
PSHE   Personal Social and Health Education
PSI   Policy Studies Institute (London)
PSIS   Personal Spine Information Service
PSL   period of study leave (GPs can apply in accordance with
   paragraph 50 of the Statement of Fees and Allowances for
   financial assistance in connection with a period of study leave to
   undertake postgraduate education, which will result in benefit
   to the GP, primary care in particular and the NHS)

PSM Professions Supplementary to Medicine
PSNC Pharmaceutical Services Negotiating Committee
(represents chemists in negotiations with the DoH)
PSNCR Public Sector Net Cash Requirement
PSND Public Sector Net Deficit
PSNI Pharmaceutical Society of Northern Ireland
PSRCS Police Standard Radio Communication System
PSS Personal Social Services
PSSRU Personal Social Services Research Unit
PSU Prescribing Support Unit
PSX Public Service Expenditure
PT part-time
PTCA percutaneous transluminal coronary angioplasty
PTL Patient Targeting List
PTS Patient Transport Services
PTSD post-traumatic stress disorder
PU prescribing unit (developed to take account of elderly patients'
greater need for medication; patients over 65 count as 3 PUs
and those under 65 as one)
PUNS patient's unmet needs
PVC prime vendor contract
PVS persistent vegetative state
PWLB Public Works Loans Board
PYE part-year effect

Q

QA quality assurance
QAA Quality Assurance Authority
QABME Quality Assurance of Basic Medical Education
QALY quality adjusted life year
QC quality control; quick connect
QCA Qualifications and Curriculum Authority
QMAS Quality Management and Analysis System
QOF Quality and Outcomes Framework
QOL quality of life
QR quick release
QSW Qualified Social Worker
QUANGO quasi-autonomous non-governmental organisation

R

R&D research and development

R&S recruitment and selection

RA regional advisor; Regional Assembly; research associate; revenue account; rheumatoid arthritis

RA(SG) Revenue Account (Specific Grants)

RAB Resource Accounting and Budgeting

RADAR Royal Association for Disability and Rehabilitation

RAE Research Assessment Exercise

RAFT Regulatory Authority for Fertility and Tissue

RAG Research Allocation Group (NHS Executive)

RAGE Radiotherapy Action Group Exposure

RAM Risk Allocation Matrix

RAO Referral and Advice Officer (first point of contact for inquiries about Social Services)

RAP Referrals, Assessments and Packages of Care in Adult Personal Social Services

RAPt Rehabilitation for Addicted Prisoners Trust

RARM Remote and Rural Medicine

RARP Resource Allocation Resource Paper

RASP Resource Allocation and Service Planning

RATE Regulatory Authority for Tissue and Embryos

RAWP Resource Allocation Working Party (the working party devised a method of distributing resources to health authorities equitably in relation to need, which was used from 1977 to 1989; the system has been superseded by weighted capitation payments)

RB Representative Body (BMA)

RBAC role-based access control

RBE relative biological effectiveness

RBMS Referral Booking and Management System

RCA root cause analysis; Royal College of Anaesthetists

RCC Rural Community Council

RCCO revenue contributions to capital outlay

RCCS Reid Clinical Classification System; revenue consequences of capital schemes

RCGP Royal College of General Practitioners

RCH Residential Care Home

RCM Royal College of Midwives

RCN Royal College of Nursing

RCO Refugee Community Organisations

RCOG Royal College of Obstetricians and Gynaecologists

RCOphth Royal College of Ophthalmologists

RCP   Royal College of Physicians
RCPath   Royal College of Pathologists
RCPCH   Royal College of Paediatrics and Child Health
RCPE   Royal College of Physicians of Edinburgh
RCPHIU   Royal College of Physicians Health Informatics Unit
RCPiLab   Royal College of Physicians Information Laboratory
RCPSG   Royal College of Physicians and Surgeons of Glasgow
RCPsych   Royal College of Psychiatrists
RCR   Royal College of Radiologists
RCS   Royal College of Surgeons
RCSE   Royal College of Surgeons of Edinburgh
RCSLT   Royal College of Speech and Language Therapists
RCT   randomised control trial
RCU   Regional Co-ordination Unit
RDA   Regional Development Agency; Rural Development Area
RDBMS   Relational Database Management System
RDC   Rural District Council (obsolete except in former UK
  colonies); Rural Development Commission
RDF   Resource Description Framework
RDN   Resource Discovery Network
RDPGPE   Regional Director of Postgraduate General Practice
  Education
RDRD   Regional Director of Research and Development
RDS   respiratory distress syndrome
RDSU   Research and Development Support Unit
RDU   Regional Dialysis Unit
REA   Regional Education Adviser
REACH   Research and Education for Children in Asthma; Retired
  Executives Action Clearing House
REAL   Research, Education, Audit, Libraries
REC   Racial Equality Council; Research Ethics Committee
REDG   Regional Education and Development Group
RES   Regional Economic Strategy
RFA   Requirements for Accreditation (GP computers)
RFC   request for comment
RFDS   Royal Flying Doctor Service
RG   Registrar-General
RGD   Revenue Grants Distribution
RGD(RG)   Revenue Grants Distribution (Review Group)
RGN   Registered General Nurse
RGPEC   Regional General Practice Education Committee

RHA   Regional Health Authority (obsolete)
RHB   Regional Hospital Board (obsolete)
RHI   Regional Head of Information
RHV   Registered Health Visitor
RIDDOR   Reporting of Injuries, Diseases and Dangerous Occurrences Regulations
RIG   Radiologically inserted gastrostomy (feeding tube)
RINN   recommended international non-proprietary name
RIPA   Royal Institute of Public Administration
RIPHH   Royal Institute of Public Health and Hygiene
RIS   Radiology Information System
RITA E   Extended RITA
RITA   Record of Individual (In-training) Training Assessment
RIU   Regulatory Impact Unit
RJDC   Regional Junior Doctors Committee
RLG   NHS Regional Librarians Group
RLQ   right lower quadrant
RLS   restless legs syndrome
RM   resource management
RMA   refuse[s] medical assistance
RMC   Regional Manpower Committee (obsolete)
RMI   resource management initiative
RMN   Registered Mental Nurse
RMO   Resident Medical Officer; responsible medical officer
RN   Registered Nurse
RNCC   Registered Nursing Care Contribution
RNHA   Registered Nursing Home Association
RNIB   Royal National Institute for the Blind
RNID   Royal National Institute for Deaf People
RNMH   Registered Nurse for the Mentally Handicapped
RO   NHS Regional Office; revenue out-turn
ROC   Retained Organs Commission (obsolete); return on capital
ROCE   return on capital employed
ROCR   Review of Central Returns
ROE   Regional Office for Europe (WHO)
ROS   return on sale
ROSPA   Royal Society for the Prevention of Accidents
RoW   Rights of Women
RP   Reporting Party
RPC   Regional Planning Conference (often now part of Regional Assembly)

RPGD Regional Postgraduate Dean
RPHTF Regional Prison Health Task Force
RPPG Regional Policy Planning Guidance
RPSGB Royal Pharmaceutical Society of Great Britain
RR relative risk
RRMS relaxing and remitting multiple sclerosis
RS Rescue Squad
RSC Royal Society of Chemistry
RSCG Regional Specialised Commissioning Group
RSCN Registered Sick Children's Nurse
RSH Royal Society of Health
RSI rapid sequence induction; repetitive strain injury; Rough Sleepers Initiative
RSIN Rural Stress Information Network
RSM Royal Society of Medicine
RSS Royal Statistical Society
RSU Regional Secure Unit; Rough Sleepers Unit
RSVP Retired and Senior Volunteers Programme
RSW Residential Social Work
RTA road traffic accident
RTF Regional Task Force
RTIA Receipts Taken Into Account (part of capital control framework)
RVSN Regional Voluntary Sector Network
RxList Internet Drug Index

S

SABA supplied air breathing apparatus
SAC Specialist Advisory Committee (of the Royal Colleges) (oversee higher medical training)
SACDA Scottish Advisory Committee on Distinction Awards
SACN Scientific Advisory Committee on Nutrition
SAD seasonal affective disorder
SAED semi-automatic external defibrillator
SaFF *Service and Finance Framework* (document setting out commissioning intentions for the following year)
SAGNIS Strategic Advisory Group for Nursing Information Systems
SAHC Scottish Association of Health Councils
SALT speech and language therapist
SAMH Scottish Association of Mental Health

SAMM Safety Assessment of Marketed Medicines (guidelines)

SAP Single Assessment Process

SAPHE Self-assessment in Professional and Higher Education (1996–99)

SAR search and rescue; subjective analysis return

SARS severe acute respiratory syndrome

SAS Scottish Ambulance Service; Staff and Associate Specialists; standard accounting system; Supplier Attachment Scheme

SASM Scottish Audit of Surgical Mortality

SAT Service Action Team

SAZ Sport Action Zone

SBS Small Business Service

SBU Swedish Council on Technology Assessment in Health Care

SCA Supplementary Credit Approval (part of capital control framework)

SCBA self-contained breathing apparatus

SCBU Special Care Baby Unit

SCCD Standing Conference on Community Development

SCD sickle cell disease

SCF Safer Communities Fund; Save the Children Fund; Scottish Council Foundation

SCG Specialised Commissioning Group

ScHARR School of Health and Related Research (University of Sheffield)

SCHIN Sowerby Centre for Health Informatics at Newcastle

SCI Self Certificate for first week of an Illness

SCID severe combined immune deficiency

SCIE Social Care Institute for Excellence

SCIEH Scottish Centre for Infection and Environmental Health

SCM Specialist in Community Medicine

SCMH Sainsbury Centre for Mental Health

SCMO Senior Clinical Medical Officer

SCODA Standing Conference on Drug Abuse

SCOPE Society for People with Cerebral Palsy

SCOPME Standing Committee on Postgraduate Medical and Dental Education

SCORPME Standing Committee on Regional Postgraduate Medical Education

SCOTH Scientific Committee on Tobacco and Health

SCP Shared Care Protocol; Short Course Programme; single capital pot; Society of Chiropodists and Podiatrists; Spinal

Column Point (position on pay-scale); Surgical Care Practitioner

SCPMDE Scottish Council for Postgraduate Medical and Dental Education

SCR Social Care Region; Summary Care Record

SCS Senior Civil Service

SCT supervised community treatment; Society of County Treasurers

SCVO Scottish Council for Voluntary Organisations

SCVS Scottish Council for Voluntary Service

SDA Service Delivery Agreement; Severe Disability Allowance (obsolete); Sex Discrimination Act

SDO Service Delivery Organisation

SDP Service Delivery Practice (NHS web database); Sub-Divisional Partnership; Severe Disability Premium

SDS Spine Directory Services

SDU service delivery unit

SEA significant event audit

SEAC Spongiform Encephalopathy Committee (advises HMG on BSE)

SEACAG South East Ambulance Clinical Audit Group

SEC Specialist Education Committee; Standards and Ethics Committee

SEG socio-economic group

SEHD Scottish Executive Health Department

SEMI severe and enduring mental illness

SEN special educational needs; State Enrolled Nurse

SEO Society of Education Officers

SEPHO South East Public Health Observatory

SERNIP Safety and Efficiency Register of New Interventional Procedures run by the Medical Royal Colleges

SERPS State Earnings Related Pension Scheme

SEU Sentence Enforcement Unit; Social Exclusion Unit

SFA Statement of Fees and Allowances (the GP's Red Book)

SFDF Scottish Food and Drink Federation

SFF *Service and Finance Framework* (document setting out commissioning intentions for the following year)

SFI Social Fund Inspector; Standing Financial Instructions (financial procedures and framework for the Health Authority)

SG staff grade

SG1 (2; 3)   Sector Group 1 etc. (part of CLP covering best value)

SGHT   Standing Group on Health Technology

SGML   Standard General Mark-up Language

SGPC   Scottish General Practitioners Committee (part of the BMA)

SGR   Scientists for Global Responsibility

SGUMDER   Standing Group on Undergraduate Medical and Dental Education and Research

SHA   Socialist Health Association; special health authority; strategic health authority

SHACE   Strategic Health Authority Chief Executive

SHACIO   Strategic Health Authority Chief Information Officer

SHAPE   Strategic Health Asset Planning and Evaluation

SHARE   Scottish Health Authorities Revenue Equalisation

SHAS   Scottish Health Advisory Service

SHEPS   Society of Health Education and Health Promotion Specialists

SHIFT   Substitution of Hospital and other Institutional-focused Technology

SHMO   Senior Hospital Medical Officer

SHO   Senior House Officer (obsolete)

SHOT   serious hazards of transfusion

SHOW   Scottish Health on the Web

SHRINE   Strategic Human Resources Information Network

SHTAC   Scottish Health Technology Assessment Centre

SI   Statutory Instrument

SIA   Spinal Injuries Association

SIDS   sudden infant death syndrome

SIFT   Service Increment for Teaching (cash to hospitals for training medical students)

SIFTR   Service Increment for Teaching and Research (the costs of undergraduate medical and dental education and research in teaching hospitals is met through SIFTR; it is intended to prevent some NHS trusts being at a disadvantage in cost terms by having to include these elements in contract prices)

SIG   special interest group

SIGN   Scottish Intercollegiate Guidelines Network

SIMS   Standardised Incident Management System

SING   Sexuality Issues Network Group

SIS   Statistical Information Service (run by IPF); Supplies Information Service

SISTC Selection into Surgical Training Centres
SITF Social Investment Task Force
SLA Service Level Agreement
SLI specific learning incident
SLIPS Safety and Leadership for Interventional Procedures and Surgery
SLS Selected List Scheme (for drugs which are restricted to particular conditions)
SMA spinal muscular atrophy
SMAC Standing Medical Advisory Committee
SMART specific, measurable, attainable, relevant, timed (of objectives)
SMAS Substance Misuse Advisory Service
SMC Scottish Medicines Consortium (a sort of Scottish NICE)
SMI severe mental impairment (people with SMI do not have to pay Council Tax)
SMO Senior Medical Officer
SMP Statutory Maternity Pay
SMR standardised morbidity ratio; standardised mortality ratio
SN staff nurse
SNAFU situation normal, all fouled up
SNMAC Standing Nursing and Midwifery Advisory Committee
SNOMED Systematised Nomenclature of Human and Veterinary Medicine
SNP Scottish Nationalist Party; single nucleotide polymorphism (a marker of genetic difference)
SNTN Scottish National Training Number
SO Standing Orders
SOAP Shipley Ophthalmic Assessment Service
SOCITM Society of Information Technology Managers
SODoH Scottish Department of Health (obsolete)
SofS Secretary of State
SOHHD Scottish Home Office and Health Department (obsolete)
SON Statement of Need
SOP Standard Operational Procedure
SoS Secretary of State
SOSIG Social Science Information Gateway
SP strategic plan
SPA Scottish Prescribing Analysis; Small Practices Association; structured professional activities
SPAIN Social Policy Ageing Information Network

SPC Summary of Product Characteristics
SPfIT Southern Programme for IT
SPG (NHS) Security Policy Group
SPIN Sandwell Public Information Network
SPP Statutory Paternity Pay
SpR Specialist Registrar
SPRAT Sheffield Peer Review Assessment Tool
SPS Standard Payroll System
SpT Specialist Trainee
SPV special purpose vehicle; Statement of Personal Values
SQC Service Quality Committee
SQP suitably qualified person
SR Senior Registrar (obsolete); Sister; Society of Radiographers;
  Spending Review
SRB Single Regeneration Budget
SRD State Registered Dietician
SRE Sex and Relationship Education
SRG Stakeholder Review Group
SRSAG Supra Regional Services Advisory group
SS spreadsheet
SSA Standard Spending Assessment
SSAP Statement of Standard Accounting Practice (now being
  replaced by FRS)
SSARG Standard Spending Assessment Reduction Grant
SSAT Social Security Appeal Tribunal
SSC Sector Skills Council; Shared Services Centre
SSCF Safer and Stronger Communities Fund
SSD Social Services Department
SSDP Strategic Service Development Plan
SSHA Society of Sexual Health Advisers
SSI Social Services Inspectorate Transferred to Commission for
  Social Care Inspection 2004; Standard Spending Indicator
  (part of SSA)
SSIP Strategic Service Implementation Plan,
SSIS Social Services Information System
SSM Special Study Module; System Status Management
SSP Statutory Sick Pay; Sub-regional Strategic Partnership
SSR Service Strategy and Regulation
SSRADU Social Services Research and Development Unit
SSRG Social Services Research Group
SSSI Site of Special Scientific Interest

STA   Specialist Training Authority of Royal Colleges

STAR   Short Term Assessment and Rehabilitation Team (social services teams which provide up to four weeks of care for people leaving hospital and residential homes and returning home)

STAR-PU   Specific Therapeutic Group Age-Sex Related Prescribing Unit

StBOP   Shifting the Balance of Power

STC   Specialty Training Committee (of local postgraduate dean)

STEIS   Strategic Executive Information System

STEP   Surgeons in Training Education Programme

STG   Special Transitional Grant (DoH money given to Social Services to change to Community Care; now defunct)

StN   Student Nurse

STP   short-term programme

StR   Specialty Registrar

STR   Structured Training Report

STrAP   Speciality Training Assessment Process (sometimes STRAP)

STSS   Short Term Support Services (planned residential respite care for people with learning disabilities)

SU   Strategy Unit (Cabinet Office); Students Union

SUI   serious untoward incident

SURE   Service User Research Enterprise

SUS   Secondary Uses Service

SWAG   Specialist Workforce Advisory Group (a group focused on the number of doctors required to provide the service)

SWG   Service Working Group; Settlement Working Group; Specialty Working Group

SWOT   An analysis of strengths, weakness, opportunities and threats (usually relates to organisations but could apply equally to an individual)

T

T&CS   terms and conditions of service (*see also* TCS)

T&O   Trauma and Orthopaedics

TAB   Team Assessment of Behaviour

TAG   Technical Advisory Group

TALOIA   there's a lot of it about

TAP   Trainee Assistant Practitioner

TATT   tired all the time

TBA to be announced; to be arranged
TC total communication; Town Council
TCBL Temporary Capital Borrowing Limit (part of capital control framework)
TCI to come in
TCP Total Commissioning Project
TCS terms and conditions of service (*see also* T&CS)
TDHC The Doctors Healthcare Company
TEACCH Treatment and Education of Autistic and Related Communication Handicapped Children
TEC Training and Enterprise Council (obsolete)
TEETH tried everything else, try homoeopathy
TEL Trust Executive Letter
TICK teamwork, integrity, courage, knowledge
TIE Theatre In Education
TIP Trust Implementation Plan (Scotland)
TIS Technical Information Services
TLA three-letter abbreviation (acronym like this one)
TMB too many birthdays
TME total managed expenditure
TME Trust Management Executive
TNA training needs analysis
TOD took own discharge
TOIL time off in lieu
TOPRA The Organisation for Professionals in Regulatory Affairs
TOPS Termination of Pregnancy Service
TOPSS Training Organisation for Personal Social Services
TPC Teenage Pregnancy Co-ordinator
tPCTs Teaching PCTs
TPD Training Programme Director
TPP Total Purchasing Project
TPQ Threshold Planning Quantity
TPU Teenage Pregnancy Unit
TQM total quality management
TR Technical Release (term used by Audit Commission)
TRBL Temporary Revenue Borrowing Limit (part of capital control framework)
TRiP Turning Research into Practice
TRIPS Trade Related Intellectual Property Rights
TRO time ran out
TSC Technical Sub-Committee

TSE Transmissible Spongiform Encephalopathies
TSG Transport Supplementary Grant
TSO The Stationery Office (formerly HMSO)
TSP Training Support Programme
TSS Total Standard Spending
TSSU Theatre Sterile Supplies Unit
TtT Train The Trainers (sometimes as TTT)
TUBE totally unnecessary breast examination
TUPE Transfer of Undertakings (Protection of Employment) Regulations 1981
TV transfer value
TWG Technical Working Group

U

UA Unitary Authority (a council which carries out all the functions in its area)
UASC unaccompanied asylum-seeking children
UASSG Unlinked Anonymous Surveys Steering Group
UB Unemployment Benefit (now JSA)
UCAS Universities College Admission Service
UEL upper explosive limit
UEMS European Union of Medical Specialists
UGM Unit General Manager
UKADCU UK Anti-Drugs Co-ordination Unit (formerly Drugs Co-ordination Unit)
UKAN United Kingdom Advocacy Network
UKCC United Kingdom Central Council for Nursing, Midwifery and Health Visiting (abolished 2002); UK Cochrane Centre
UKCHHO UK Clearing House on Health Outcomes (Leeds)
UKCRC UK Clinical Research Collaboration
UKCRN UK Clinical Research Network
UKDIPG UK Drug Information Pharmacists Group
UKHFAN UK Health for All Network
UKOLN The UK Office for Library and Information Networking
UKPFO The UK Foundation Programme Office
UKPHA UK Public Health Alliance
UKTSSA UK Transplant Support Service Authority
UKXIRA UK Xenotransplantation Interim Regulatory Authority
ULC unit labour cost (staff cost required to provide a given unit of activity)
ULTRA Unrelated Live Transplant Regulatory Authority

UMLS Unified Medical Language System
UNICEF United Nations Children's Fund
UNISON Trades Union for public sector workers, incorporating COHSE, NALGO and NUPE
UPA Underprivileged Area (a measure of deprivation; 0 is the mean for England)
URL Universal (or Uniform) Resource Locator (on Internet)
UTD Unit Training Director
UTG Unified Training Grade (now SpR)
UTH University Teaching Hospital

V

VA voluntary action; voluntary-aided; Vote Account
VAMP a GP information system supplier user group
VB Volunteer Bureau
VC variable cost; voluntary-controlled
VCO(s) Voluntary and Community Organisation(s)
VCS Voluntary and Community Sector
VCT Voluntary Competitive Tendering
VDRFAMP Vascular Disease Risk Factor Assessment and Management Process
VFM value for money
VFMU Value for Money Unit
VHI Voluntary Health Insurance (Ireland)
VOCOSE Voluntary, Community and Social Economy
VPE Virtual Private Exchange (type of internal telephone network)
VSA volatile substance abuse
VSC Voluntary Service Co-ordinator
VSNTO Voluntary Sector National Training Organisation
VSO Voluntary Sector Option (New Deal); Voluntary Service Overseas
VSPG Voluntary Sector Policy and Grants
VSpR Visiting Specialist Registrar
VTE venous thromboembolism
VTN Visiting Training Number
VTR Vocational Training Record
VTS Vocational Training Scheme (the mandatory scheme of structured experience and training in hospitals and the community for doctors planning a career in general practice)

W

WAA Working Age Agency
WADEM World Association for Disaster and Emergency Medicine
WAHAT Welsh Association of Health Authorities and Trusts
WAIS wide area information server
WAN wide area network
WAT Workforce Action Team
WBA workplace-based assessment
WCH Wales Centre for Health
WCVA Wales Council for Voluntary Action
WDC Workforce Development Confederation
WeBNF web-accessible BNF
WEST Winter and Emergency Services Team
WF Work Foundation (formerly Industrial Society)
WFP Working for Patients
WFTC Working Families Tax Credit (now replaced by Tax Credits)
WGSMT Working Group on Specialist Medical Training
WHCSA Welsh Health Common Services Agency (obsolete; now part of Welsh Health Estates)
WHDI Welsh Health Development International
WHE Welsh Health Estates
WHO World Health Organization
WiC Walk in Centre
WIGS women in grey suits
WIH work in hand
WIMS Works Information Management System
WIsH Welsh Innovations in Healthcare
WIST Women in Surgical Training Scheme
WM workload measure (e.g. OBD, LOS, FCE)
WMA World Medical Association
WMQI West Midlands Quality Observatory
WNAB Workforce Numbers Advisory Board
WNC Women's National Commission
WO Welsh Office
WONCA World Organisation of National Colleges Academies and Academic Associations of General Practitioners/Family Physicians
WP White Paper; word processor
WP10 Working Paper 10 (now NMET)
WPA Western Provident Association

WPBA workplace-based assessments
WRC Women's Resource Centre
WRT Workforce Review Team
WRVS Women's Royal Voluntary Service
WTC Working Tax Credit
WTD Working Time Directive
WTEP whole time equivalent posts
WTEs whole-time equivalents (the total of whole-time staff, plus the whole time equivalent of part-time staff, which is obtained by dividing the hours worked in a year by part-timers by the number of hours in the whole-time working year)
WTI Waiting Time Initiative
WU Women's Unit

Y

YCS young chronic sick
YDU Young Disabled Unit
YHYCYS *Your Health, Your Care, Your Say*
YOT Youth Offender Team

Z

ZBB Zero-Base Budgeting